STRENGTH TRAINING UNLEASHED

A Guide for Gym Goers, Athletes, and Seniors

JETO-RIVAR SANON

© Copyright Jeto-Rivar Sanon 2023 - All rights reserved.

The content contained within this book may not be reproduced, duplicated or transmitted without direct written permission from the author or the publisher.

Under no circumstances will any blame or legal responsibility be held against the publisher, or author, for any damages, reparation, or monetary loss due to the information contained within this book. Either directly or indirectly. You are responsible for your own choices, actions, and results.

Legal Notice:
This book is copyright protected. This book is only for personal use. You cannot amend, distribute, sell, use, quote or paraphrase any part, or the content within this book, without the consent of the author or publisher.

Disclaimer Notice:
Please note the information contained within this document is for educational and entertainment purposes only. All effort has been executed to present accurate, up to date, and reliable, complete information. No warranties of any kind are declared or implied. Readers acknowledge that the author is not engaging in the rendering of legal, financial, medical or professional advice. The content within this book has been derived from various sources. Please consult a licensed professional before attempting any techniques outlined in this book.

By reading this document, the reader agrees that under no circumstances is the author responsible for any losses, direct or indirect, which are incurred as a result of the use of the information contained within this document, including, but not limited to, — errors, omissions, or inaccuracies.

Table of Contents

Introduction 1

Chapter 1: Unleash the Power of Strength Training 7

Chapter 2: Power Up Your Gym Game 26

Chapter 3: Strength Training for Athletes 48

Chapter 4: Empowering Aging Warriors with Intense Strength Training 63

Chapter 5: Nourishment for Optimal Regeneration 80

Chapter 6: Mind-Muscle Connection and Mental Toughness 106

Chapter 7: Tracking your Gains 129

Conclusion 140

Introduction

The concept of strength training is based on the idea of conquering resistance. This resistance can be provided by the weight of external items (for example, dumbbells) that must be moved (lifted, pushed, or pulled) or by the weight of the body itself, which must be held or lifted in various positions. Strength exercise helps to stabilize the metabolism, strengthens the bones, muscles, tendons, and ligaments, improves anaerobic endurance, benefits the nervous system, and trains the cardiovascular system. There are many things that can affect how much muscle you have. For example, the type of exercise you do could affect how much muscle you have.

What concerns do you have regarding strength training? You may believe that your body is too weak or not used to exercising. Unless you have been advised otherwise by a medical practitioner based on a specific condition or injury, you shouldn't avoid exercising. According to studies, exercising can really reduce your risk of falling. Regular exercise improves not only the stability, balance, and flexibility of your body but also the strength of your bones. Are you worried about osteoporosis or brittle bones? One of the most effective strategies to build strength is to engage in regular physical activity. Even if you think it's too late to start exercising, you'd be wrong.

Adults are responsible for their own health and well-being. For them, the best way to maintain good health and fitness is through regular physical activity. Numerous age-related health problems might be staved off with regular physical activity. Maintaining fitness is critical since it aids in the growth of your muscles. In this way, you can carry out daily tasks without relying on anyone. Always establish a schedule for physical activity. If you are unable to exercise consistently, at the very least, try to do so on some days during the week, as any physical activity is preferable to none.

Maintaining a healthy lifestyle throughout our lives increases our chances of remaining healthy as we age. Experts assure us that individuals who have lived a sedentary lifestyle can benefit from beginning a regular fitness plan at any age.

It makes no difference if you are 30 or 60 or whether you have been active or idle throughout your life. This book will demonstrate how to change your body and life regardless of who you are or your current level of health and fitness. Exercise not only strengthens the body but also aids in memory retention and dementia prevention. Additionally, it might assist you in keeping your freedom and way of life. Maintaining strength and agility allows you to keep doing the things you enjoy and lessens the chance that you will need help.

Growing older and/or living a sedentary lifestyle has its own set of challenges. Cognitive and physical declines, as well as social changes, might result in loneliness, incapacity, and depression in certain individuals. Mobility and agility gradually diminish as we age, making ordinary tasks more challenging to execute. If you're having similar problems, strength-training exercises might help you get back on your feet and take charge of your life.

If you want to maintain your health and vitality, now is the time to act. While it is undeniable that maintaining strength and muscle tone is simpler for an 18-year-old person than it is for a 40-year-old person, strength and muscle tone can be maintained and even enhanced throughout life. That is encouraging news. The bad news is that as you age, your body changes.

According to studies, over 60% of working-age adults do not engage in any form of physical activity on a regular basis. Additionally, many of these adults remain inactive during both leisure and work hours. Because this age group has historically been at a higher risk for cardiovascular disease and other health problems as a result of insufficient physical activity, it is critical for them to engage in some type of exercise or strength training on a consistent basis. To maintain your health as you age, ensure that your weekly plan includes a minimum of moderate aerobic exercise and strength training. To get the above-mentioned benefits, all you need to do is add these types of exercises to your daily workouts.

Regular physical activity will have a significant positive impact on your overall health. Not only that, but it will also help you maintain an increased level of energy throughout the day. Another benefit of regular physical activity is improved heart health, particularly when strength-training exercises are performed correctly. Strength training routines work your heart, arms, and legs all at the same time. This leads to increased oxygen intake by the muscles, which benefits the cardiovascular system.

Strength training also aids in the toning of the abdomen and other muscle areas. This will reduce your chance of falling and give you more joint flexibility. Having more muscle mass increases the number of calories you burn during exercise. As a result, your body fat percentage will also be reduced. Being physically active not only aids in weight loss but can also help you keep your bones strong and improve your overall health. Regular strength training activities help to increase the calcium content of the bones, making them less susceptible to osteoporosis later in life.

Strength training can aid in the prevention of cognitive illnesses affecting the brain as people age, such as Alzheimer's and dementia. Regular physical activity helps senior citizens and people who live a sedentary lifestyle enhance their mood and overcome anxiety and sadness. It's also good for your mental health if you do a lot of strength training because you'll be able to deal with stress better later in life.

Strength training is critical for reducing the aging process due to the benefits it provides. Cardiovascular health is critical for people of all ages because it can play a critical role in preventing strokes, one of the major causes of death in modern times. Physical activity and strength training activities help to enhance cardiovascular function and minimize the risk of heart disease and high blood pressure, which are both extremely frequent health problems. Most significantly, frequent strength training improves the efficiency of your heart, which results in a longer lifespan. This book will give gym-goers, athletes, and seniors a detailed plan for strength training as well as talk about how to add it to their workouts without putting their health at risk.

Regular strength training will improve your body's efficiency and make buttoning your favorite pants a little easier. You do not have to make drastic life adjustments to have a stronger core and gain the associated benefits. By the end of this book, you will know how to strengthen your core muscles, keep your balance, and maintain your mobility. These are tools that you can use again and again.

Developing a stronger, more capable physique is not nearly as difficult or as hard as most people believe. Just a few hours a week for a few months is enough to make a difference. To attain outstanding results, you do not need a plethora of various exercises, expensive gym equipment, or intricate moves. The true science behind reversing age-related muscle loss and rebuilding your body is straightforward and far simpler than the majority of people believe. You have the ability to transform your body and your life, no matter who you are.

Consider waking up each morning with a sense of anticipation, knowing that your body is now cooperating with you rather than against you. Consider feeling more capable and secure in your body and being prepared to take control of other areas of your life. Think about being able to achieve all of your goals without being held back by a lack of energy. You may have all of these things, and obtaining them is simpler than you believe.

You do not have to make drastic life adjustments to have a stronger core and gain the associated benefits. This guide is for anyone interested in learning more about strength training. This book covers everything. There are detailed explanations of a wide range of exercises and programs, as well as information on the fundamentals of strength training (such as technique, nutrition, and program design). This book is a helpful resource for athletes, gym rats, and elderly citizens who want to get stronger and fitter because of its emphasis on both athletic performance and general health.

Please check with your physician before beginning any of the workouts in this book if you have any health concerns. Having stated that, let's work together to make your life healthier and more enjoyable. Excellent, let us begin!

Chapter 1

Unleash the Power of Strength Training

Introduction to Strength Training Principles

These are the pillars upon which any good strength training program is built:

- The overload principle says that the musculoskeletal system needs to be overworked over time to get the adaptive response from strength training and keep it. This keeps the muscles from getting used to their new normal and keeps the adaptive response from strength training going.

- The principle of specificity states that adaptations occur only in trained muscles.

- To get the best results, overloading should happen at the right level and at the right time. This is done through progression or periodization.

- Uniqueness. Because people react differently to training stimuli, everybody needs a unique set of instructions.

- Removing the stimulus that prompted the training can reverse its effects.

Equipment for Strength Training

Examples of many forms of strength training include:

- Free weights, including barbells, dumbbells, and kettlebells, are the traditional strength training tools.

- Weighted balls or bags, such as sand ones

- Weight machines are machines with adjustable seats and handles that are connected to weights or hydraulics.

- Resistance bands offer resistance when stretched. They're easy to transport and modify for a wide variety of exercises. As you move, the bands' resistance stays the same.

- Suspension equipment lets people work out using only their own body weight and the force of gravity.

- Your own body weight is ideal for squats, push-ups, and chin-ups (particularly useful when traveling or at work).

Creating a Strength Training Routine

Paying close attention to safety and form can help keep you out of harm's way. The most important factors to think about when developing an exercise routine are:

- Choice
- Order
- Frequency
- Intensity
- Volume
- Rest interval
- Progression

The emphasis of the exercise should be on

- Strength
- Hypertrophy
- Power
- Muscular Endurance.

Benefits of strength training:

- Build up your bone density. The risk of osteoporosis can be decreased through the use of strength training to promote bone density.

- Take control of your weight. Increased calorie expenditure and the maintenance or reduction of excess fat are two of the many benefits of strength training for health and fitness.

- Improve the standard of living. Research shows that doing strength training regularly can improve both your physical and mental health, making you happier with your life. The joints are another important body part that strength training can help safeguard. In addition to improving your balance, strength training may also make you less likely to experience injuries from slips, trips, and falls. As you get older, this can help you keep your freedom.

- Control ongoing medical issues. A variety of chronic diseases and their associated symptoms can be alleviated via regular strength training.

- A number of studies have found that frequent strength training and aerobic exercise can benefit older individuals' cognitive functioning and ability to learn new information.

Consider the options:

Depending on your goals, you can either train at home or at a gym. Options include:

- Work on your muscle strength at home or at the gym. Common options could be:

- The individual's total mass. Many forms of exercise can be performed with minimal or no apparatus at all. You can also do lunges, squats, push-ups, and pull-ups.

- Resistance tubing. Resistance tubing provides resistance when it is stretched, and it does so at a low price and with a low weight. These days, you can pick up a resistance tube at almost any sports goods store or go online and find a wide variety of options.

- Free weights. Traditional strength training equipment includes barbells and dumbbells. Soup cans will do in the absence of actual weights at home. The use of medicine balls and kettlebells are two further alternatives.

- The use of weightlifting equipment. Many kinds of resistance machines are available at most gyms. Household weight machines are also available for purchase.

- Exercises utilizing suspension cables. Exercising while suspended from a cable is another choice. As an alternative to traditional forms of weight training like push-ups and planks, cable suspension training suspends a body component, like the legs, while the rest of the body is worked out using only body weight.

Getting started

- Talk to your doctor before beginning a strength training or aerobic fitness program if you have a chronic ailment or are over the age of 40 and haven't been active lately.

- Do some light cardio, such as brisk walking, for five to ten minutes before starting your strength training session. Cold muscles are more prone to injury.

- Select a weight or amount of resistance that will leave you fatigued after 12 to 15 repetitions. Increase the weight or resistance of a workout only when you feel ready to take on more reps.

- There is evidence to suggest that for most people, a single set of 12–15 repetitions with a suitable weight can be just as effective for muscle growth as three sets of the same exercise. To build muscle, you need to exhaust the muscle you're training until you just can't do another repetition. If you start to feel fatigued at a higher number of reps, you are probably using a smaller weight, which will make it simpler to keep your technique steady.

- You should wait a full day between targeting individual muscle groups to allow for recovery.

- Listen to your body for cues as well. Stop doing a strength training activity if it hurts. Think about going lighter or waiting a few days before trying again.

- Strength training can cause injuries if not done correctly. If you're new to strength training, it's important to acquire proper form and technique from a trainer or fitness expert. Don't forget to take deep breaths when you strength train.

Weight Training: The Basics

FITT refers to a set of components that work together to make weight training effective.

- Frequency of training: How often do you train?

- The intensity of training: How strenuous your training sessions are

- Time spent: Duration of the session

- Type of Exercise: Which Exercises

Muscles and Movements

When it comes to building muscle, knowledge of how your muscles function is crucial.

Two distinct types of muscular contractions exist:

- Isometric contractions: When performing an isometric contraction, the muscle stays at its resting length throughout the movement. One illustrative action is pushing against a wall.

- Isotonic contractions: During isotonic contractions, the muscle alternately contracts and relaxes. The "concentric" contraction is the one that results in a shorter length, whereas the "eccentric" contraction results in a longer length.

The muscle contracts during the concentric portion of the movement (raising the dumbbell) and relaxes during the eccentric portion (lowering the dumbbell), as in a dumbbell arm curl. Eccentric contractions are typically the cause of muscle pain.

Joint Movements

Joint motion is related to muscular contractions. The four most common joint motions are flexion, extension, abduction, and adduction.

- A joint is said to be flexed when the angle between its two ends decreases. In an arm curl, the upward motion reduces the elbow joint angle.

- Extension is the opposite of flexion because it involves making the angle bigger while making the weight smaller.

- A sideways motion away from the body's midline is called abduction. Raise one leg out to the side as an illustration.

- When a body part is adducted, it is brought closer to the body's midline.

Muscle Groups

Briefly, the major muscle groups are the arms, shoulders, chest, back, legs, buttocks, and belly. You can exercise in a variety of ways that focus on different muscle groups.

- Exercising at a high intensity for short bursts, like in high-intensity interval training (HIIT) or CrossFit, is one way to work your complete body in a single workout.

- Body part split training is a common part of traditional bodybuilding routines. On one day, you work on one muscle group, and on the next day, you work on a different muscle group.

- You can train your main muscle groups by concentrating on the "major lifts," such as the squat, bench press, deadlift, clean and jerk, and snatches.

Reps, Sets, and RM

You should be familiar with the following workout terminology:

- One squat, chin-up, or arm curl counts as one repetition (rep).
- The number of repetitions you do without resting is called a set. We'll say that one set of arm curls consists of ten reps.
- The rest period is the time between sets.
- Your one-repetition maximum (ORM) is the most weight you can lift in a single workout. Therefore, your 12-repetition maximum is your absolute maximum strength.

Example: When the barbell is set to 40 pounds, it takes 60 seconds to do three sets of twelve reps at maximum effort.

That's three sets of twelve arm curls at maximum intensity with a weight of forty pounds, with a minute of rest in between each set. The question now is how to calculate the appropriate number of repetitions, sets, and breaks in between them. In general, the process looks like this: The specifics are something you and your coach can work on.

- Weight, reps, and rest periods are all optimized for strength training.

- Hypertrophy is the process of getting bigger muscles by doing fewer sets with fewer reps and less rest between sets.

- Strength endurance is less important now, and there are more repetitions and even less time to rest.

- Lighter weights and longer rests, with an emphasis on lifting velocity, characterize power training.

These are some broad guidelines. You can find your optimal workout by experimenting with different sets, reps, rest periods, and exercise types.

Example: Bench press exercise plans can vary widely from person to person, but here are some examples based on a hypothetical starting weight of 160 lb (73 kg):

Bench Press - 1RM = 160 pounds

1. Strength: 140 pounds, 2 X 5, 180 seconds
2. Hypertrophy: 120 pounds, 3 X 10, 60 seconds
3. Strength Endurance: 100 pounds, 3 X 15, 45 seconds
4. Power: 90 pounds, 3 X 8, 120 seconds

One thing to keep in mind is that resting sufficiently between heavy sets is essential for optimal outcomes during strength training. Each rep needs to be performed at a very high explosive velocity for power training to be effective, so a suitable rest interval is also crucial. When building muscle and explosive power, it's essential to allow for adequate recovery time between sets. But shorter intervals are better when training for hypertrophy and strength endurance, though they are not required.

Speed of Exercise Execution

Another thing that affects how well an exercise works is the rate at which it is done. This is called the contraction velocity. Some broad recommendations for weightlifting objectives are provided below.

- Strength: 1-2 seconds concentric and eccentric
- Hypertrophy: 2-5 seconds concentric and eccentric
- Endurance: 1-2 seconds concentric and eccentric
- Power: less than 1 second concentric, 1-2 seconds eccentric

Calculating 1RM

The United States National Strength and Conditioning Association suggests the following theoretical distribution of repetitions in relation to a percentage of your one-repetition maximum (1RM), which is your maximum lift, using 160 pounds as an example:

- 100% of 1RM: 160 pounds —1 repetition
- 85% of 1RM: 136 pounds — 6 repetitions
- 67% of 1RM: 107 pounds — 12 repetitions
- 65% of 1RM: 104 pounds — 15 repetitions
- 60% of 1RM: 96 pounds — warmup reps

This means that for any given exercise, you should be able to do one rep at your maximum effort, six reps at 85 percent of your maximum effort, and fifteen reps at 65 percent of your maximum effort in a single set. Don't use this as gospel; instead, use it as a guide to help you figure out what weights will give you the best results.

Building Strength

The overload principle is used to increase muscle strength, growth, and endurance. That means you'll have to start out light and gradually build up your strength as you go. Training the neuromuscular system and the interplay between the nerves and muscles is what develops strength, as opposed to training muscle morphology, size, and constitution, which leads to hypertrophy. When building muscle, it's important to use heavy weights and rest for extended times between sets. Muscle growth does increase strength, but not necessarily to the same degree as strength training does. Strength training can include anywhere from three to six repetitions at maximum effort, with more advanced lifters able to handle loads of one to three repetitions.

Increasing muscle size

When building muscle, hypertrophy training typically involves more sets with less weight and less rest in between them than strength training. This training directly leads to changes in the body's metabolism that make it easier to gain weight. Hypertrophy training can help you gain strength, but if you want to compete in bodybuilding or powerlifting, you need to have very specific goals. Most people who lift weights for reasons other than competition are trying to strike a balance between strength and muscle growth by following a weight training program. Microtrauma and subsequent healing are a key part of the muscle-building process.

Muscle fibers undergo microscopic trauma when under stress; these tears are healed, and the muscle is rebuilt stronger once the athlete rests. At the cellular level, progress can sometimes feel like going backwards before advancing again. There's significant debate about whether or not larger muscle fibers (cells) are the sole cause of muscle growth or if the formation of new cells also contributes to muscle development. During hypertrophy, the number of myofibrils, which are the parts of a muscle that contract, goes up. The sarcoplasmic reticulum, which is the fluid-filled space around a muscle cell, also gets bigger. Most hypertrophy training consists of 2–5 sets of 8–12 repetitions done at 70–80% of one's maximum effort.

Building muscle endurance

Intense sets of reps are used to hone muscle endurance. For instance, focusing on 15-20 reps per set rather than strength or hypertrophy is what local muscle endurance training is all about. Although the gains in strength and hypertrophy won't be as big as with higher-intensity programs, they'll still be better than doing nothing at all, and the gains in aerobic fitness can be substantial. When building muscle endurance, a range of 15-20 reps per set is optimal. Typically, three sets are performed. However, you should consider whether or not you could be better off using your time by training in a skill-based sport, such as running, swimming, or bicycling.

Building muscle power

Given that power is the rate at which labor is accomplished, time is an essential component. Your strength increases if you can perform the same exercise faster than your companion. Increasing the repetition speed of the lifts is a key component of power training. Weight training for sports like football, where strength, bulk, and speed are valued, benefits from the concept of power. When exercising for power, it is best to start with a modest weight and work up to heavier ones as your strength increases. The American College of Sports Medicine suggests lifting 30–60% of one's one-repetition maximum and resting for 2–3 minutes in between sets.

Frequency and overtraining

Your training frequency and intensity should be based on your goals, experience, age, health, fitness, and other criteria, including the availability of training resources and time. Your trainer or coach should think about all of these things and come up with a plan that works for you. The delicate balancing act of weight training is between stimulating muscles and the neurological system, adapting to new demands, and recovering. Overtraining syndrome happens when a person trains too quickly and reaches an abnormally high level.

For beginners, training three times per week is ideal for making steady progress; however, some may find that training twice per week is more manageable. Most experts tell beginners who are just starting out to wait at least 48 hours between weight training sessions. Six days a week of training is common for experts and professionals, though many also use split systems, which involve training various muscle groups on different days.

Types of Exercises

For a beginner, choosing from among the hundreds of exercises designed to strengthen certain muscles and muscle groups might be a daunting task. Machines, free weights, racks and frames, workouts involving only the body, bands, balls, and many more provide a wide range of options. Aerobic and strength training, as well as exercises that focus on specific muscles or fitness goals, fall into this category.

- Compound exercises. working for multiple muscle groups at once. When training many big muscle groups at once, as is commonly the case with compound exercises, more than one joint is used. Squats, deadlifts, seated cable rows, and lat pulldowns are all great examples.

- Isolation exercises. Practicing by oneself. One definition of an isolation exercise is a movement pattern that emphasizes the use of only one joint and a single muscle group. The biceps curl with dumbbells and the quadriceps extension machine are two good examples.

Here are 7 different strength-building techniques to help you reach your full potential.

Agile strength

The capacity to swiftly and forcefully change one's course of action typifies agile strength. This permits the body to move in any chosen direction with relative ease and fluidity. Coordination and balance are enhanced, and the risk of injury is reduced. Maybe you don't even realize it, but you're probably constantly improving your agility and strength. Consider how many times you've had to carry a heavy purse, shopping cart, or child car seat through a store, your house, or up a flight of stairs.

Agility in the workplace

Multidirectional, light-to-moderate weight training is indicative of agility. Exercises like medicine ball lat shuffles and direction-change sprints are recommended by experts. Perform farmer's carries with a weight that is moderately heavy for 30 to 60 seconds at a time. Try it out by walking or jogging in circles around your house or the gym, and then rely on your sense of touch to tell you when to switch gears. You should do three to five sets with a minute or two of rest in between.

Endurance strength

How long you can keep going is the ultimate test of endurance. When compared to the typical HIIT routine, this one is the polar opposite. Keeping moving forces the body to use both aerobic and anaerobic pathways, which can improve long-term postural stability and aerobic capacity in the muscles.

Work on endurance strength as follows:

It's best to begin your strength training with only your body weight and then progress to using weights as your strength increases. Professionals advise doing three to five rounds of 15 squats and 10 push-ups in a row with minimal rest in between. You'll find that you're able to return to work faster and sooner after injuries as your strength and endurance increase.

Explosive strength

Strength training with high-intensity intervals (HIIT) focuses on developing explosive strength for powerful, rapid movements. The recruitment of motor units, intramuscular coordination, response time, and muscular and connective tissue resilience are all enhanced. Activities like jumping and lifting weights are examples of ways to work out hard for a short amount of time.

How to work explosive strength:

Focus on explosive exercises like box jumps, snatches, and cleans. An excellent warmup exercise is throwing a medicine ball. Do five sets of forceful chest-to-wall throws without stopping, and then take a break. If you want to win the next round, you need to either throw with more force or move backwards a bit and keep trying to build up to that kind of intensity in your throws. Complete five sets of five reps.

Maximum strength

How much weight you can lift with one hand is a good indicator of your maximum strength. In addition to boosting hormone levels responsible for muscular growth, increasing bone density, and strengthening the muscles, these routines also help generate the fast-twitch muscle fibers necessary for producing powerful, explosive movements. Since bone density naturally declines with age, this is particularly crucial in preparing the body for the aging process.

How to work at maximum strength:

The goal of this exercise is to perform a few sets with a hefty weight. Heavy squats, deadlifts, bench presses, hip thrusts, and powerlifting are some of the activities recommended by fitness professionals for gauging one's true strength. Due to the increased risk of injury associated with lifting heavier weights, well-planned programs should be adhered to in order to avoid overtraining and ensure adequate rest and recovery between workouts.

Speed strength

Put simply, your speed is directly proportional to your speed strength. It works more muscles, leading to better muscular balance, and it increases flexibility by putting your muscles through a wider range of motion. Training in this manner can shorten the time it takes for muscles to go through a full cycle of lengthening and contracting, hence improving reaction times and athletic performance.

How to Increase Work Speed and Strength

Sprinting is the simplest approach to improving your speed. You can experiment with interval training on your own or follow a coach-led program.

Starting Strength

With no prior momentum, starting strength is the initial burst of power required to get going. The capacity of muscle and connective tissue to generate more force, move faster, and rise from a seated position can all benefit from this. Making your muscles, bones, and joints stronger through exercise is crucial to your well-being.

How to work at starting strength:

Since "starting strength" refers to the force with which an action is initiated, these are the kinds of workouts in which you must rapidly increase your intensity from zero to sixty. The experts say that dead-start kettlebell swings, sprinter jumps, and sit-down squats are all fantastic methods to work it.

Relative strength

The development of relative strength, which accounts for an individual's body composition, follows the improvement of the other six modalities. Relative strength is a measure of an individual's strength in comparison to their body size, and it is commonly observed that smaller people have more relative strength. If you want to know how strong you are in comparison to others, record your maximum repetitions on a given bodyweight exercise and divide that number by your weight. You'll be able to accomplish more reps as time goes on since your strength will increase.

How to work with relative strength:

Relative strength is developed alongside the other types of strength listed above; hence, it is difficult to specifically train it. You can increase your relative power by shifting your attention to the other modalities.

Chapter 2

Power Up Your Gym Game

Strength training has a variety of health advantages.

Makes you stronger. When you regularly engage in strength training, you increase your muscle mass and strength, making it easier to carry out daily chores and enhancing your sports performance. It's useful for endurance athletes since it helps them keep their muscle mass while training for longer periods of time.

Burns calories efficiently. When you do strength training to gain muscle mass, your resting metabolic rate goes up, and you burn more calories for up to 72 hours after the workout.

Decreases abdominal fat. Consistently carrying extra weight around the middle is associated with a higher chance of developing serious conditions such as diabetes, cancer, non-alcoholic fatty liver disease, and heart disease. It has been established that strength training can aid in the reduction of abdominal fat as well as overall weight.

It can help you appear leaner. By increasing your muscle mass and decreasing your body fat, you can improve your appearance. As muscle is more dense than fat, it takes up less volume in the body. Muscle definition, resulting in a stronger and slimmer appearance, is another benefit of reducing body fat and increasing muscle mass.

Decreases your risk of falls. Studies show that seniors over 65 who took part in a fitness program with resistance training, balance exercises, and functional training were 34% less likely to fall.

Lowers your risk of injury. By enhancing muscle and tendon strength and flexibility, strength training can lessen the likelihood of injury. In addition to lowering the injury risk for both young and old athletes, strength training is also useful for correcting musculoskeletal imbalances. One meta-analysis found that the risk of injury went down by 4% for every 10% increase in the amount of strength training.

Improves heart health. Regular strength training is good for your health in many ways, like keeping your weight steady and keeping your blood sugar levels normal.

Promotes healthy glucose control. By improving insulin sensitivity and decreasing blood sugar levels, strength training can aid diabetics in better managing their condition. Research on people who regularly did strength training showed that their risk of getting type 2 diabetes went down by 30%.

Improves flexibility and range of motion. Joint range of motion (ROM) is improved through strength training, which in turn improves mobility and flexibility. Because stretching has the same effect on a range of motion, it's crucial to work up to a full range of motion in each exercise without sacrificing form.

Boosts your self-esteem. Confidence can be boosted through strength training since it teaches you to face adversity head-on, achieve success, and value your own abilities. Strength training has been linked to positive body image, attractiveness, body satisfaction, and social anxiety about one's appearance. It has also been linked to a good self-image, physical strength, and physical self-worth.

It makes your bones stronger. Strength training is essential for bone development because it sends a signal to bone-building cells to produce stronger bones, which is important for preventing osteoporosis, fractures, and falls. Nobody is too old to accomplish this.

Boosts your mood. The benefits of strength training extend beyond just physical health. Studies have shown that it can improve mental health in general by elevating one's mood and sense of pride in one's abilities. Endorphins are chemicals that can make you feel happier. When you exercise, these chemicals are also released.

Improves brain health. Working out the muscles may have a positive effect on the processing speed, memory, and executive function of the elderly. It also makes more brain-derived neurotrophic factor (BDNF) and reduces inflammation and blood flow, which are both good for the brain.

Encourages a higher standard of living. Researchers have found that strength training improves health and longevity. Research has shown that resistance training has far-reaching benefits for physical and emotional well-being as well as pain management, general health, and vitality. Arthritis sufferers may also benefit from strength training to improve their quality of life.

Building a Strength Routine: The Essential Guide

Learn how to create and stick to a strength training plan that is specific to your needs.

Creating your very own strength training program may be a lot of fun because it allows you to tailor your efforts to your specific needs and interests. You can use these as a starting point for developing your own approach and sticking to it.

Pick three tangible goals

In order to get started on your plan, choose three measurable goals. Ideally, they would be actions that could be evaluated initially and ultimately. Setting measurable goals, such as a certain amount of weight lifted or a certain number of reps completed, makes it much simpler to track improvement and change training accordingly.

Evaluate your schedule

Look at your schedule and decide how often you will be able to exercise and how much time you will have for each session. Aiming for three to four strength-based workouts each week is ideal, since this provides the body with sufficient time to rest and recuperate while building muscle. If three to four days of strength training each week is too ambitious, pick a schedule you can realistically keep for at least 90% of the time and build on that.

Design your workouts

The first step in designing effective workouts is figuring out your goals and time constraints. To supplement your deadlift training, pick one main lift (for example, a deadlift) and then a few accessory movements to go along with it. Selecting a single lift as your primary focus throughout each session will help your body hone its strength in that area. Put together enough of these workouts for a week or two. You should continue doing the same exercises you did for the first two weeks for at least another two months. It will help your muscles get stronger at certain movements and give you a good way to track your improvement.

Stick to it!

Now that you have a plan, think about how you'll stick to it. Keeping a record of your workout's weight and number of repetitions will help you stay on track and hold yourself accountable. Set aside the time for your workouts just as you would for a crucial business meeting, and you'll be far more likely to keep that commitment. Finally, have an expert review your fitness level before beginning a new strength training program. Your chances of being hurt will go way down, and you'll be able to safely and effectively gain muscle.

Routines for the Entire Body That Produce Real Results

Full Body Training Notes

In contrast to training splits, full-body regimens have a few distinct advantages. You will be working all of your major muscle groups every day of training, but with fewer sets per body part each day. Training your whole body at once can be incredibly hard. Be strong against the temptation to tack on extra training sessions. Here are a few other details to keep in mind concerning total-body workouts:

- **Training Frequency.** There are typically three full-body workouts per week on Mondays, Wednesdays, and Fridays. You should never train your entire body on consecutive days.

- **Exercise Selection.** Heavy compound lifts are a staple of full-body workouts. You may stimulate muscle growth without performing a large number of exercises for each body region if you focus on mastering a small number of main lifts.

- **Minor muscle groups.** There are typically not a lot of isolated exercises that target smaller muscle groups. It's important to push through the feeling that your back delts, forearms, abs, etc. aren't getting a decent enough workout if you're concentrating on working out your entire body. By performing compound lifts three times a week, you are effectively targeting the entire body. The smallest of muscle groups will react to this method.

- **Mental Connection.** Some gym-goers have trouble making the mental leap to full-body workouts. Some people can start to doubt their decision to forego split training if they observe everyone else doing it. Keep in mind that the lifters of yesteryear didn't necessarily lack knowledge just because they relied on full-body routines. For many, many years, full-body workouts were the norm.

The Muscle and Strength 5x5 Routine for the Whole Body

Building muscle and strength with the Muscle & Strength 5x5 is as easy as following a simple regimen. Aim to increase your strength by focusing on a select few exercises each training day. Stay true to how the program is supposed to be used and don't make any changes to it. This routine's emphasis on core lifts is key to building both strength and muscle mass. By improving your performance on these lifts, you can coerce your body into growing in size. Don't forget to take in a healthy amount of calories. If followed correctly, this routine will do wonders for slim males looking to bulk up and gain strength.

- **Training Level** - Beginner.

- **Target Group** - heavy lifters who want to bulk up quickly. You can use it to prepare for more difficult full-body exercises or to just build up your strength.

- Every week (Monday, Wednesday, and Friday).

- **Routine Duration**- four to six months. If you've been doing this and seeing great results so far, you should feel free to keep at it for as long as you like.

Monday

Exercise	Sets	Reps
Squat	5	5
Bench Press	5	5
Wide Grip Pull Up	3	10
Weighted Sit Up	3	10-20

Wednesday

Exercise	Sets	Reps
Deadlift	4	5
Seated Barbell Press	5	5
Barbell Curls	3	5-10
Seated Calf Raise	3	10-25

Friday

Exercise	Sets	Reps
Front Squat	5	5
Close Grip Bench Press	5	5
Bent Over Row	5	5
Romanian Deadlift	5	5

Notes for the Muscle and Strength 5x5 Workout:

- **5x5 Sets.** Two functional warm-up sets are included in each 5x5 set. The working weight for the remaining three sets is 60% of what you used for the first set. The weight for your second set should be 80 percent of what you lifted for the final three repetitions.

- **3 Set Exercises.** "3 sets" does not include the warm-up set for an exercise. If you feel it's necessary or prudent, do some warming up.

- **Rest.** Two-minute breaks should be taken between exercises. You can take as much as five minutes off between deadlift and squat sessions.

- **Deadlifts.** The 4x5 deadlifting program consists of one "working" heavy set and three warming sets. In the first set, you'll do 5 repetitions at half your heavy set weight. On your second set, choose a weight that is 70 percent of what you used for your heavy set and complete 5 repetitions. For the third set, you will perform five reps at 90 percent of the weight you used for the heavy set.

Train your entire body with 20 reps of squats at a high load and moderate resistance.

The 20-Rep Squat HLM Full-Body Exercise is an alternative method of increasing muscular mass. You will be performing squats on Monday and Friday, with Monday being the heavier of the two. One set of 20 squats will be completed on Friday. This is an extremely challenging set that yields superb outcomes. Those who have reached a plateau with their muscular gains using traditional training splits and are ready for a drastic change should try this full-body program. On Mondays, you'll be putting in some serious work at the gym by way of straightforward, heavy compound motions. On Wednesdays, you'll be doing less intense workouts with more repetitions. On Fridays, you'll be doing medium-intensity work with rep ranges of 8–12 for predominantly big compound exercises.

- Training Level - Beginner +.

- Target Group - If you are attempting to shock your body and pack on muscle but are a beginner or intermediate lifter, you should try. You'll benefit greatly from participating in this program.

- Every week (Monday, Wednesday, and Friday).

- Routine Duration - If the results you are getting from this method are stable, keep at it.

Monday

Exercise	Sets	Reps
Squat	3	3-5
Deadlift	1	5
Bench Press	3	3-5
Seated Barbell Press	3	3-5

Wednesday

Exercise	Sets	Reps
Leg Press or Leg Extension	2	15
Dumbbell Flys or Weighted Chest Dip	2	15
Lat Pull Down or Wide Grip Pull Up	2	15
Leg Curl	2	15
Dumbbell Lateral Raise	2	15
Skull Crushers or Cable Tricep Extension	2	15
Concentration Curl or EZ Bar Preacher Curl	2	15
Seated Calf Raise	2	15
Rear Laterals	2	15

Friday

Exercise	Sets	Reps
Squat	1	20
Dumbbell Bench Press	3	6 to 10
Bent Over Row	3	6 to 10
Romanian Deadlift	2	6 to 10
Seated Dumbbell Press	3	6 to 10
French Press or Close Grip Bench Press	2	6 to 10
Barbell Curl or Dumbbell Curl	2	6 to 10
Standing Calf Raise	2	6 to 10

The full-body exercise consists of 20 reps of squats. Notes:

- **20 Rep Squat.** It's possible that you won't be able to complete a full set of 20 reps of squats until several weeks have passed. Exercise patience and select a starting weight that is on the lower end of the scale. Put yourself to the test and see if you can increase the weight on the bar by five pounds once every week or two.

- **Light Day.** Daytime workouts should be difficult without becoming impossible. You should try to push yourself as much as possible and lift heavier weights.

- **Heavy Day.** You should progress to the next weight level when you can execute three sets of five reps with the same weight on the bench press, seated press, or squat. Every other week, add 5 pounds to your deadlift, or 10 pounds in a month. If you find that you can't do 5 reps every set, you should drop the weight by 10 pounds for your next workout.

- **Medium Day.** Challenge yourself toward the middle of the day, but don't overdo it. If you're doing multiple sets of an exercise, keep the weight constant. When you get to 10 reps throughout all sets, that's when you go up in weight by 5.

- **Deadlifts.** Get in three sets of warm-ups before tackling your single training set. Start your workout with 5 repetitions using 50% of your heavy set weight. When performing your second warm-up set, aim for 5 repetitions at 70% of your heavy set weight. On your third warm-up set, you'll use a weight that's 90% of your heavy set and perform 5 repetitions.

- **Rest.** Two-minute breaks should be taken between exercises. While switching between squats and deadlifts, take a break of at least 1 to 2 minutes between each set.
- **Warm-up Sets.** Warm-ups are not included in the listed sets. Start each of the exercises cold.

The Grind is a Total-Body Strength Training Routine.

The Grind isn't as terrible as it sounds, I promise. It's a fantastic method for gaining muscle mass without putting undue stress on the body. The idea is straightforward: in order to make progress in each of the major lifts, you should prioritize sets with fewer repetitions, with the goal of increasing your rep total by exactly one. If you do The Grind for a year, you can increase your strength by 75–100 pounds in the bench press, deadlift, and squat. This is the ideal exercise routine for someone who has achieved significant progress and needs to keep the ball rolling. Although the primary goal is to increase strength, the program is also beneficial for someone seeking to increase muscle mass with supplementary activities.

- **Training Level** - Intermediate weightlifter: a beginner with significant strength gains and a firm understanding of proper technique.
- **Target Group** - Bodybuilders and strength athletes that wish to speed up their muscle and strength growth.

- Three days a week (Monday, Wednesday, Friday)
- **Routine Duration -** If you are seeing steady improvement, by all means, stick with the regimen.

Monday

Exercise	Sets	Reps
Squat	6	2-3
Romanian Deadlift	2	6-10
Barbell Rows	3	6-10
Weighted Chest Dip	2	6-10
Seated Dumbbell Press	2	6-10

Wednesday

Exercise	Sets	Reps
Bench Press	6	2-3
Front Squat	3	6-10
Pull Up	3	6-10
Barbell Curl	2	6-10
Weighted Sit Up	2	10-25

Friday

Exercise	Sets	Reps
Deadlift	6	2-3
Seated Barbell Press	3	6-10
Close Grip Bench Press	3	6-10
Seated Calf Raise	2	10-25
Dumbbell Side Bends	2	8-15

The Grind is a full-body workout that includes the following notes:

- **Squat, Deadlift and Bench Press.** Weight should be added until six sets of three repetitions have become routine. No more than three reps should be done in a set.

- **Rest.** Between each set, take a break of around 2 minutes. If you're doing squats and deadlifts, you might need as much as a five-minute break between sets.

- **Warm-up Sets.** Sets that were used for warming up are not counted. Prepare for each activity on the list by performing the necessary warm-up.

The Full-Body Exercise Based on the Quick Start A/B Format

The Quick Start A/B Workout is a great addition to full-body workouts, and it is especially good for people who haven't worked out much or at all before. There is an emphasis on heavy lifting, but direct training for the traps, calves, and abs is also included. Squatting and deadlifting will make up a significant portion of your workouts as you try to improve your overall strength. If you're having trouble gaining muscle mass with more traditional bodybuilding splits, the Quick Start A/B is the regimen for you. The repetition range of 8–10 between sets makes this workout an effective method for gaining muscle.

- **Training Level** - Someone with some training experience and a firm knowledge of the proper form for the key lifts would be an excellent fit at this level.

- **Target Group -** Those who are having trouble gaining weight using traditional bodybuilding split programs are referred to as "hard gainers" or "underweight lifters."

- Every week (Monday, Wednesday, and Friday). Every other day, you'll switch between two different physical activities. The first week is A/B/A, and then week 2 is B/A/B.

- **Routine Duration -** Keep at it for 6 months or as long as you're seeing steady improvement.

Workout A

Exercise	Sets	Reps
Squat	4	8-10
Bench Press	4	8-10
Barbell Row	4	8-10
Military Press	4	8-10
Seated Calf Raise	2	10-20
Weighted Sit Up	2	10-20

Workout B

Exercise	Sets	Reps
Deadlift	2	10-15
Leg Press	2	12-15
Incline Dumbbell Bench Press	4	8-10
Dumbbell Shrug	4	8-10
Barbell Curls	4	8-10
Standing Calf Raise	2	10-20
Hanging Knee Raise	2	10-25

The Full-Body Exercise Based on the Quick Start A/B Format Notes:

- **Progression.** Keep in mind that growth is especially important for the hard gainer. As soon as you reach a point where you can complete 10 reps in a set, increase the weight. Put in more effort during each set, but avoid going to the point of exhaustion.

- **Rest.** Two-minute breaks should be taken between exercises. Depending on your form, you may require as much as 5 minutes of rest in between sets of deadlifts and squats.

- **Warm-up Sets.** Warm-ups are not included in the listed sets. The listed exercises should be preceded by the proper warm-up.

Intermediate Full-Body Workout for Muscle and Strength

If you're an intermediate lifter who's utilized split routines in the past but wants to try something new, this is the routine for you. To begin with, while your body adjusts to being worked on three times weekly, you may need to utilize smaller weights. Refrain from increasing your volume too much every day. Full-body routines already involve about as much work per muscle group per week as split routines.

- **Training Level** - Intermediate.

- **Target Group** - Skilled bodybuilders interested in trying out natural methods.

- Three Days A Week (Monday, Wednesday, Friday)

- **Routine Duration** - Keep at it for 6 months or as long as you're seeing steady improvement. Adjustments to suit your unique requirements and body type will become second nature with time.

Monday

Exercise	Sets	Reps
Squat	3	6-15
Bench Press	3	6-10
Pull Up or Lat Pull Down	3	6-12
Leg Curl	3	8-15
Upright Row	2	6-10
Skullcrusher	2	6-10
Barbell Curl	2	6-12
Barbell Shrug	2	8-15
Ab Exercise	2	10-25

Wednesday

Exercise	Sets	Reps
Deadlift	3*	5-10
Leg Extension	3	8-15
Dumbbell Bench Press	3	6-10
Seated Barbell Press	3	6-10
Seated Calf Raise	2	10-20
Cable Tricep Extension	2	6-12
Concentration Curl	2	6-12
Rear Lateral	2	8-15
Ab Exercise	2	10-25

Friday

Exercise	Sets	Reps
Leg Press	3	10-20
Barbell Row	3	6-10
Romanian Deadlift	2	6-10
Incline Bench Press	3	6-10
Side Lateral	2	8-15
Close Grip Bench Press	3	6-10
Pinwheel Curl	2	6-12
Dumbbell Shrug	2	8-15
Ab Exercise	2	10-25

An intermediate full-body exercise for building muscle and strength:

- **Rep Ranges.** The representativeness ranges are presented as examples only.

- **Weight.** Since you'll be making 9 different moves every day, it's recommended that you stick with a consistent weight throughout. Workout times will be reduced as a result.

- **Progression.** Pay attention to your form and make sure you're progressing with each set. Put your preferred method of progression into effect.

- **Rest.** In between each set, you should take a 2-minute break. It's possible that you'll require as much as 5 minutes of rest in between sets of deadlifts and squats.

- **Warm-up Sets.** The listed sets are exclusive of warm-ups. Do the necessary warm-ups before beginning any of the exercises on the list.

- **Deadlifts.** There is only one intense set that you will be required to complete. Choose a weight that is 60% of your heaviest set and perform 5 repetitions. In your second set, you will perform 5 repetitions at 80% of the weight you used in your last heavy set. A heavy set is the third set of a set.

How to Get Rid of a Plateau: Step-by-Step Instructions

Getting Rid of and Preventing a Plateau

You can eliminate a plateau by following these steps, which can be used either to avoid a plateau or to break through one.

Take Adequate Rest. Relaxation and rehabilitation are crucial for any gym goer, but especially so for those who have hit a stalemate. Taking a break from working out for a week to ten days can do wonders, allowing you to return to your routine feeling refreshed and ready to give it your all. Instead of wasting your free time zoning out in front of the TV and stuffing your face with junk food, try doing something enjoyable, entertaining, and useful instead.

Eat Enough Quality Food. If you've hit a weight-loss or muscle-gain plateau, it might be time to reevaluate your calorie demands, break down your macros, and upgrade to healthier fare. If you're constantly hungry, it's a symptom that you're not getting enough to eat. Protein needs, such as 1 gram of protein per pound of body weight, must be met daily.

Switch Up Your Routine. The human body is a marvelous creation, able to effortlessly adjust to any conditions it encounters. Muscle gain is best accomplished by varying your workout schedule every 4 to 6 weeks. Altering the sequence in which you complete your exercises or performing them in a different order are both viable options for achieving this goal. Don't be afraid to mix things up, play around, and keep things interesting.

Stay FIT. The workouts you perform and the way you perform them should both be adjusted. The acronym FIT refers to frequency, intensity, and time. These are priceless bits of wisdom for pushing past a rut. They are adaptable to one's current cardio- and strength training regimen. Let's just go over these:

- Modifying your workout schedule's frequency

- Workout intensity refers to how hard or easily you are pushing yourself during your workouts.

- Train for different amounts of time.

Get Enough Sleep. Muscle gain and fitness, in general, require not just regular exercise and a nutritious diet but also sufficient rest each night. For optimal performance during the day, adults need 7 to 8 hours of sleep every night. If you want more energy and better results from your workouts, sleep more.

Keep Workouts Under an Hour. Lifting weights is meant to encourage growth, not stunt it. However, overtraining, especially if it continues for a long time, can cause muscle deterioration. Hormones that aid in growth reach their peak within the first 30 minutes after exercise and then begin to diminish. Never train for more than an hour and fifteen minutes at a time.

Challenge Yourself. Muscles expand and harden in response to overload, so it's important to keep pushing yourself if you want to keep seeing gains. When you exercise, it's important to keep track of how many repetitions and how many sets you perform for each activity. Next, when you repeat that exercise routine, give yourself a harder task:

- Maintain your current set count, but add one or two repetitions to each set.
- Alternate between sets and keep reps at their current levels.
- You can increase the weight if you keep the reps and sets the same.

Don't Over Do It. You need to take a rest. Particularly after a strenuous workout, it's best to wait a few days before re-working the same muscle area. Overuse and fatigue will weaken your muscles if you don't get enough rest.

If you want to develop muscle, be sure to take it easy on the cardio. If your goal is to gain muscle, you should limit your aerobic workouts to 20 to 30 minutes at a time and perform them no more than three to four times per week. Cardiovascular exercise for a long time can hurt testosterone levels and the body's ability to build muscle.

Chapter 3

Strength Training for Athletes

Knowing the fundamentals of sports-specific strength training

All aspects of human behavior have undergone gradual change over time. Let's use throwing as an example because it's a simple motor skill. Historically, the ability to throw was crucial for survival in both the hunt and the defense. While throwing is no longer a central part of these sports, it is nevertheless widely used in a variety of other sports (e.g., athletics, baseball, handball, etc.). A primitive hunter's job required pinpoint accuracy in order to successfully bring down prey and get a meal.

Training for a sport with rules is done with the intention of improving one's performance in that sport, be it at the individual or team level. No task can be completed with optimal efficiency in a single day. Many factors together influence efficiency. Maximum performance in the motor skills required for a given sport is the primary goal of any athlete's training. Motor competence and motor aptitude are directly tied to the specific sport being played. A person's motor skills can be thought of as a set of internal, genetic presuppositions that are used repeatedly throughout life to perform locomotor actions.

Power, speed, stamina, coordination, and adaptability are all part of this category. Sporting prowess is the visible manifestation of one's motor ability. Skills in sports are the foundation for achieving success in a regulated sporting activity. Assumptions like this are learned mechanically. But, without inspiration, it would be impossible to practice athletic abilities or hone locomotor skills. It's generally agreed that the term "motivation" refers to an innate drive to complete a task. Tactical competence is the final component necessary for actualizing performance. Tactics refer to the methodical execution of game strategies. Individual, crucial aspects of sports training are grouped together as "training components."

- For the most part, motor skill development is the primary focus of the physical training component.

- The "technical" part of a sport refers to the practice and drills that help a person develop motor abilities.

- The tactical part of getting ready for a sport is learning and practicing different ways to play the game with a purpose.

- Psychological training improves the athlete's character.

Components of Sports Training and Their Attributes

Physical Component

The focus of physical training is on the methodical improvement of motor skills and their practical application in a chosen sporting activity. Important motor skill domains include:

- Speed abilities
- Force abilities
- Endurance abilities
- Coordinative abilities
- Flexibility

Differentiating motor skills alone isn't enough to define how an athlete's talents reveal themselves in their chosen sport. The physical demands placed on the athlete during training are most directly associated with the particular sport being pursued. Sports like the 400-meter dash and the marathon call for continuous high (in the former's case) or moderate (in the latter's case) motor task intensity. Yet, in other sports like basketball or soccer, the athlete is required to perform a wide variety of motor actions, from holding still to sprinting at full speed, with frequent directional changes. Many sports have different requirements, all of which have something to do with the athlete's physical abilities.

- The ability to generate a large amount of force in a single competitive move, such as kicking a soccer ball or jumping for a basketball (force),

- Capacity for sustained physical activity (endurance)
- Ability to run fast (speed)
- The most important parts of high-intensity training (agility) are being able to move quickly and change directions quickly.

Below, we'll get into the finer points of the many subcategories. There are five guiding concepts that should inform every aspect of a well-designed training program. Specificity, the size of the stimulus for adaptation, and progression are the three pillars that hold up all the other principles.

Specificity

There is a high degree of specificity involved in training for a given sport. The athlete learns to perform better in the actions that make up that sport's specialized subset. For instance, takeoff in a volleyball attack strike is characterized by taking off from both feet; thus, specialized exercises supporting the appropriate type of takeoff must be performed while training rapid force.

Size of the adaptation stimulus

When it comes to sports preparation, using a smaller size than the athlete is accustomed to can serve as an optimal and adaptable stimulus. Regardless of how well thought out a training program is, the athlete will not progress as far as they could if they are not exposed to the best possible adaptation stimuli. There is no correlation between exposure to subliminal stimuli and improved performance. Applying this principle can be done in a variety of ways, such as by increasing the number of exercises, the number of training sessions per week, the size of the exercise in force training, drills, or sets, the preference for complex exercises over simple ones, the reduction of rest periods between sets, or a combination of these factors.

Progression

For systematic training to yield ever-increasing gains, the training load and intensity must rise in tandem. When applied correctly, the principle of progressive increase leads to a cumulative training effect. This becomes clear when different training variables, like the number of training sessions per week, the type of exercise, the level of difficulty, etc., are changed.

Technical component

Acquiring, retaining, and imparting motor skills are important to technical education. From the perspective of sports training, motor skills can be broken down into two categories:

Humans acquire rudimentary competencies as part of their typical ontogenetic maturation. gait, run, jump, climb, do basic overhand throwing, etc. The substance of a given sports discipline serves as the foundation for developing expertise in that field. Skills in volleyball include things like setting, receiving, blocking, serving, and so on. The end goal of honing these abilities is to become highly automated.

Athletes use these skills throughout their careers at all levels of competition. This ability remains with the athlete throughout his sporting career, regardless of his level of success. Developing these abilities ought to be in line with a more holistic view of sports practice. This idea holds that regardless of the focus of a given sport's training program, it must incorporate the development of a sizable number of motor skills that are not central to that program but are nonetheless useful in achieving its overall goals. For instance, these may consist of gymnastic or athletic abilities useful for a player's rehabilitation, compensating, and all-around growth as an athlete. A person's capacity to move can be classified into three broad categories based on their motor behavior.

General versus special skills

While general agility drills focus on improving a single aspect of coordination, skill-specific drills bring all of the skills together. One such general skill that improves static balance is the ability to stand on one foot. On the other hand, balancing on one foot on a bar could be a unique skill that is shown during a gymnastics routine.

Closed versus open skills

These tasks and conditions are predetermined, making closed agility a useful skill. Examples of closed skills include gymnastic routines and figure skating sets. The assignments and conditions under "open skill" are not predetermined. The goal of the practice is to be able to quickly respond and adjust to new or unexpected stimuli and scenarios when the context shifts during the performance. When playing defense, for instance, it's common for a player to have to react quickly to an opponent's unexpected action, requiring them to draw on their wide skill set.

Continuous versus discrete versus serial skills

Tasks that can be described as "continuous" do not have a clear beginning or end. Cycling, skating, and rowing are all examples of sports with cyclical elements. There is no ambiguity about the beginning or end of a discrete task. Skills with an acyclic character structure are one example (throw, jump). Skills are layered upon one another in a sequential fashion to complete a serial activity, with the sum of the parts being the final result. The ability to throw a javelin and the ability to long jump are examples of skills that have both cyclic and acyclic parts.

Tactical component

By "tactics," we imply the application of strategy to a given racing situation. In practice, you'll draw primarily from your knowledge of potential strategies for dealing with every given racial circumstance. Within the framework of the chosen long-term vision of sports training, the rate of progress toward obtaining potential answers to race-situation challenges must be consistent with the time spent training.

Every volleyball squad has at least one area of vulnerability that the other team can exploit. Let's pretend an unknown team's roster features a player who struggles to avoid damage when taking the ball on offense. At the moment, reception is the foundation of a high-quality volleyball game. Let's further assume they have a solid setter on their roster. As a result, if a player is shorter than the rest of the court's players, it is advantageous to serve at them and try to direct the opponent's offense over the area of the net that is being defended by the shorter player.

When a service is meant to make it difficult for the receiver to see the ball, the game's tactics shift to focus on a practical solution to the problem. He'd have to take the longest route feasible to the reception area; the offensive strategy would change based on the defensive player's location, etc. Here is a synopsis of yet another possible strategic approach: Creating tension between your opponents is the foundation of a high-quality game. Thus, the strategy is to choose an opponent who has a tendency to get hot under the collar and approach him at the appropriate time.

Sports Performance Structure

Success in sports is defined as the level at which a motor task constrained by the rules of a certain activity is completed. It is generally accepted that different aspects of sports performance are mostly autonomous from one another. Several sports training experts agree on a core set of principles that apply across all sports:

- Technical factors
- Tactical factors
- Somatic factors
- Fitness factors
- Psychical factors

Somatic considerations, such as choosing taller children for volleyball and basketball and shorter ones for gymnastics, are examples of how these factors are taken into account when selecting talent. There is a direct correlation between the aforementioned sports training parameters and athletic performance antics, which are examples of how these factors are taken into account when selecting talent. There is a direct correlation between the aforementioned sports training parameters and athletic performance. The factors that affect sports performance are varied. Each sport has its own unique set of criteria, and their relative weight and order of importance might vary widely.

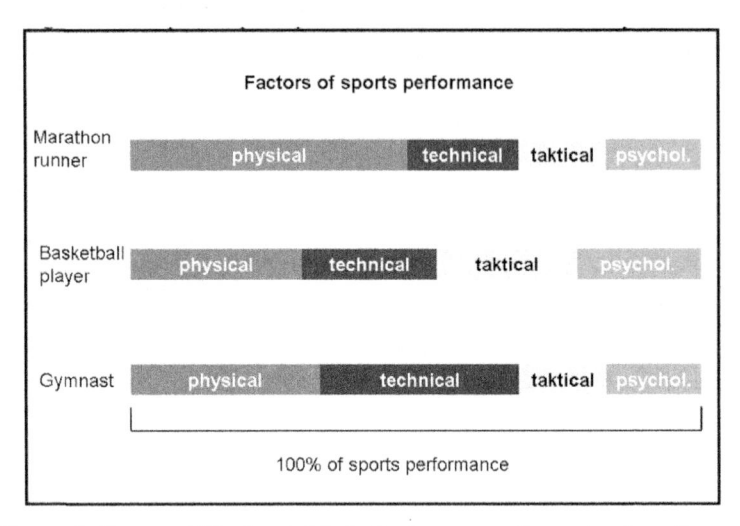

Figure 1: Factors Affecting Athletic Performance: Examples from Several Sports

While developing long-term endurance is a key aspect of the year's microcycle for marathon runners, it is less of a focus for sports gymnasts. This image provides a model of the components that influence athletic performance (Figure 2).

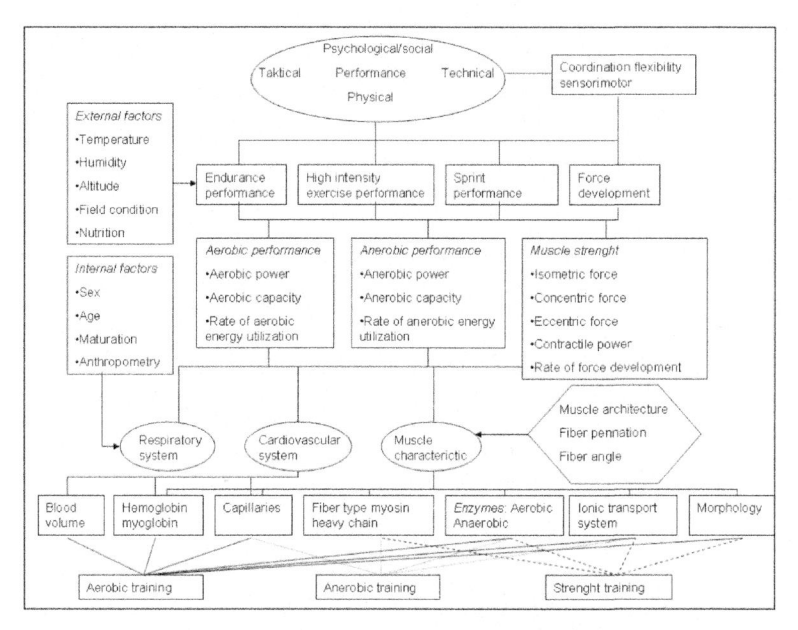

Figure 2 Here's a good illustration of a component that affects performance in sports.

As a direct result of what has been said, an athlete's performance in sports depends on his or her technical skills and psychological and social traits. There is a link between these things. For example, technical skill is limited if you don't have enough physical skill. Conversely, poor technical competence will limit the effectiveness of the tactical element. Physical requirements in sports are directly associated with the tasks that athletes are expected to complete.

Athletic prowess is based on the unique qualities of a person's respiratory and circulatory systems, muscles, and the interplay of their nervous systems. There are many different parts that make up the muscular system, and they all play a role in the muscle's mechanical and metabolic properties.

The shape, architecture, and myosin isoform composition of a muscle all have a big effect on its ability to contract, which can be measured by things like maximal isometric, concentrative, maximal rate of force development, eccentric contraction forces, and power production. The levels of glycolytic muscle enzymes and ionic transport mechanisms have a big effect on anaerobic strength and stamina. Similar to this, the amounts of mitochondrial enzymes and capillary density affect the endurance performance of muscle fibers, which in turn affects the production of force and the peak power output of human skeletal muscle. Breathing, heartbeat, and muscle strength are all affected by genes, but they can all be improved by working out. Things like the temperature, the climate, and the playing surface for outdoor sports could all have a negative impact on an athlete's performance.

Athletes can greatly benefit from strength training.

Any athlete, regardless of age or skill level, can benefit from strength training. Here are just some of the many benefits you'll reap from making strength training a regular part of your routine:

Reduce body fat, increase muscle and skeletal strength, and increase bone density. Physiologically, we know that the human body can adapt to various stresses. Muscles, tendons (the tissue attaching muscle to bone to act as energy transmission and a spring), and ligaments (which limit motion from bone to bone) may all adapt and develop stronger through regular strength training and progressive loading. In a similar vein, the right kind of force can cause the bone to become denser and stronger, a process known as osteogenesis.

By making well-targeted movement patterns, you can make your muscles, joints, and bones stronger, more mobile, and more durable.

Strength training is beneficial for young people because it boosts their overall levels of physical activity, helps them build sturdy muscle foundations, supports their growing skeletons, and instills in them a lifelong love of exercise. On the other hand, senior athletes can keep their strength and muscle mass, strengthen their bones, increase the range of motion in their joints, and stay healthy as they age to improve their performance.

Improved neuromuscular coordination and mobility.One of the first and most noticeable changes in your body when you begin a regular strength training program is improved neuromuscular function. This is when the nervous system recruits the right muscle fibers more quickly and efficiently during exercise. Improved movement efficiency and coordination can keep endurance athletes from getting tired as quickly and lower their rate of perceived exertion, which keeps them in the game longer. Strength training can cut down on the amount of energy you need to run a certain distance at a certain speed.

Increase the force output and growth rate. Producing power requires a mix of force and velocity. When we train our muscles to get stronger, we increase our body's capacity to produce force, which, in turn, allows us to apply more force at a faster rate of contraction, which in turn increases our power and explosiveness. Athletes in any discipline can benefit from a faster rate of force development; this is true for team and field sport athletes, track and field competitors, and endurance and multisport competitors like cyclists, rowers, runners, and triathletes. Power and explosiveness can be developed by performing progressive plyometric activities, such as jumps, hops, skips, and bounds, using only the athlete's own body weight or by lifting small to moderate loads (such as in Olympic weightlifting) at high velocities.

Create a "performance physique" and perfect body composition. Strength exercises that focus on the major muscle groups can boost metabolism for up to 72 hours after exercise, making them one of the finest types of exercise for promoting fat loss and achieving an appropriate body composition. Both Type 1 and Type 2 muscle fibers can grow larger with hypertrophy exercise, with the latter experiencing more growth as a result. This results in increased muscle mass and a higher basal metabolic rate. Some athletes may benefit from this extra muscular mass, while those with a slimmer build may see greater gains in performance.

Prevent injuries and prove inequalities. By building up the power of both the primary muscle groups and the supporting muscles that are crucial to the demands of the sport, strength training can be an effective prescription for lowering the likelihood of injuries. Getting this kind of muscle mass is very important for lowering the risk of overuse injuries and the muscle imbalances that come from training too hard. With regular strength training, an athlete can handle heavier loads with less risk of injury because their muscles and bones are stronger and they can move better.

As part of our regular workouts, we may develop imbalances or weak spots. These problems can be fixed by choosing the right exercises. Returning from injury often involves a period of strength training as part of the rehabilitation process, with the goal of gradually exposing the athlete to suitable loads and tasks that are sport-specific. Any of these traits can help an athlete recover and get back to their best performance, so it's important to work on them all during the rehabilitation process.

Improved Athletic Performance Through Strength Training

Fundamentals of Strength Training

While training for strength, you should lift weights that are between 60 and 100 percent of your maximum, depending on your goals. Training in this fashion not only stresses the muscles to their limitations but also places a premium on the neuromuscular system (the muscles and their connected nerves) capacity for effective muscle recruitment. Overloading, progression, specific training, tailored rest, and rest periods are the five pillars upon which strength training rests. In the right proportions, they establish the foundation for building strength and athleticism over time.

In order to overload, you need to train at an intensity that triggers microscopic microtears within the muscles. This triggers the body's adaptation mechanism. Hence, your body starts to fix the damage done by intense resistance training. Muscles get stronger as a result of this overcompensation, which is a normal part of the body's recovery process. Both strength and hypertrophy training are based on this mechanism, which is known as "supercompensation."

The term "progression" is used to describe the methodical process of continually stressing your muscles and providing them with progressively more challenging tasks in strength training. This is why the progressive overload theory of strength training is so frequently discussed among coaches and athletes. Just increasing the weight, the number of sets, or the number of repetitions will not produce noticeable gains in performance. It is also a good idea to use a variety of training methods so that the muscles are exposed to a wide range of stimuli.

The process of building muscle mass should be tailored to each individual's specific sport and ambitions. This includes both sport-specific muscle training and periodization of workouts to ensure steady improvement without risking injury. Keep in mind that your ultimate objective is to boost your own physical efficiency.

Resistance training of this intensity necessitates lengthy recovery periods. Most athletes are unaware that muscular growth and skill acquisition occur while they sleep. This is especially crucial for strength training, as your body will not be able to handle another rigorous workout for at least 48 hours. But after 72 hours, your strength levels will begin to drop again. Hence, you should incorporate gentler activities or complete rest periods between more strenuous sessions into your fitness routine.

Chapter 4

Empowering Aging Warriors with Intense Strength Training

Only a handful of the many benefits that strength training can bring to seniors are listed here.

- Muscle mass declines as you get older. In fact, by the time someone reaches the age of 70, they have typically lost 25% of their muscle mass.

- Muscle atrophy is something that can be mitigated by engaging in regular strength exercises.

- Age-related declines in metabolism may contribute to gaining weight. Weightlifting, cardiovascular exercise, and a good diet can all help mitigate this.

- Fall and fracture risks can be mitigated by engaging in strength training.

- In addition to being good for your health, regular strength training can also improve your mood.

Advice for Strength Training Better as You Age

Strength training involves a wide variety of options, such as:

- Using your own body weight for resistance
- Barbells
- Dumbbells
- Kettlebells
- Weight machines

Safe Strength Exercises for the Elderly

Always consult a physician before beginning any new workout program. Think about any health conditions or injuries that could prevent you from strength training. Also, if you are lifting more weight than you can handle, weightlifting might cause a transient rise in blood pressure. Lifting weights properly can have a beneficial influence on hypertension.

Changing how you work out is an important part of any effort to improve your health. This involves eating plenty of protein, which is essential for muscle development and repair. If you want better outcomes, cutting back on booze and cigarettes is a good place to start. Then make sure you get plenty of shut-eye to fully unwind and let your muscles recover. Listen to your body as you go through the muscle-building process. Each day will be different. Some days, you may feel worse than others. Take close notice of any discomfort and cease promptly if it persists. Do not resume exercising until the soreness has subsided. Take it slow and easy at first.

It doesn't matter how long or hard you plan to work out; warming up is always a good idea first. By doing a warm-up, you can get your heart rate up without putting too much stress on your heart and lungs. As a bonus, your muscles will receive a better oxygen supply. To get ready, give yourself about 5 minutes. Pay attention to the muscles you plan to work on that day. Shoulder rolls, toe touches, ankle circles, and marching in place are all excellent examples of warm-ups.

Weight Training Strength, flexibility, balance, and mobility can all be enhanced with consistent practice. Two days a week at a modest intensity is a good place to start, and as you feel better, you may add more days and ramp up the intensity. Three or four days a week of exercise are acceptable.

Squats

In terms of physical activity, this is arguably the most crucial for the elderly. If you can squat, you'll have more mobility and be able to do things like rise from a chair, get out of bed, pick something up off the floor, and exit a vehicle. Squats are essential for establishing a solid base in the lower body. Your other strength training will benefit from this strength as well. Your hamstrings, quadriceps, and glutes will all benefit from this movement. If you're having trouble keeping your balance, you can practice squats while holding onto a table or a wall.

1. Your feet should be hip-to shoulder-width apart, and your toes should point forward. Keep your eyes ahead of you, your feet firmly planted, your chest up, and your hips back. Make sure your knees aren't folding in and that they're

hovering directly above your ankles. Balance yourself by extending your arms in front of you. Hold a deep squat for as long as you can, ideally 1–2 seconds.

2. Go back to the starting position by pushing through your heels. At least ten times, or as many as you can.

3. Modify the squats so that they are less taxing on the knees if you have trouble with them. Put your feet on the floor and take a seat. While pushing off the chair, keep your chest up and your knees out. Go as far as is comfortable for you. The procedure must be repeated while seated.

4. To make it more challenging, you can either perform more of them, move more slowly, or use heavier weights. You can do squats with different levels of resistance when you hold a dumbbell, kettlebell, or medicine ball.

Lunges

They are crucial for building muscle in the thighs, buttocks, and hips. Lunges are great for building stability, which is essential for standing and walking. Keep your feet hip-width apart and your hands on your hips as you stand.

1. Keep your torso upright and step forward with your right foot. You should only go as far as you feel comfortable.

2. Bring your right foot back to its initial position.

3. Try it out on your left foot now.

4. You can do this ten times or as many as feels natural.

5. To make it simpler, cling to a nearby chair or railing for support.

6. Using a 2–5-pound weight in each hand, resistance can be increased.

Wall Push-Ups

For elders, this modification of the standard push-up is a great time-saver. You won't need to squat down and then fight your way back up! The emphasis of the movement is on building strength in the upper body, especially the arms and chest.

1. Place yourself about 2 feet away from a solid wall, or as close as you feel safe.

2. The best position for your hands is against the wall in front of your shoulders.

3. Bend your elbows and keep your body straight. When bending your arms, keep them close to your sides rather than jutting out.

4. Reverse direction as soon as your face touches the wall and stop.

5. Do 10 repetitions or as many as you feel comfortable with.

Step-Ups

This is a great leg exercise since it trains your body to do something that is crucial: stand up. There are a lot fewer places you can go if you can't use the stairs. The strengthening of your glutes and quadriceps through doing this balance drill will make it easier for you to ascend and descend stairs, as well as leap over obstacles. Put two to five-pound weights on each foot's ankles for an extra test of strength.

1. Stand tall at the base of the stairs. Keep your hands on the railing for balance.

2. Raise your right foot slowly and put it fully on the step.

3. Just keep putting your left foot in front of the right.

4. Take a few measured steps backward, first with your right foot and then your left.

5. Do this ten times or as often as you feel necessary.

6. You should lower yourself gradually by putting your right foot down first, then your left.

Seated bicycle crunches

Bicycle crunches are a good ab exercise because they work the abs and strengthen the core. I suggest completing movements while seated so that the elderly don't have to get up and down from the floor.

1. Take a seat on a sturdy chair and put both feet firmly on the ground. Place your hands behind your head with your elbows extended.

2. Raise your left knee until it's in line with your right elbow, then twist from the waist.

3. Just untwist it and bring it back to its original position. Be patient with yourself if you can't immediately bring your elbow to your knee. Muscle development is an iterative process that necessitates dedicated effort and patience. Just keep at it!

4. The correct move is to switch sides and bring the right knee near the left elbow.

5. Do this exercise 10 times on each side or until you feel fatigued.

Overhead press and shoulder press

This is an excellent senior-friendly dumbbell exercise. Strengthening and stabilizing the shoulders also benefits the back and the arms. It will be useful for overhead lifting. I suggest using a one-pound weight or no weight at all as a starting point. If you don't want to hurt yourself, you should ease into it. Listen to your gut instincts. The overhead press can be done while standing, sitting, or even lying down. Do not stand because you risk hurting your back.

1. While sitting tall on a chair, maintain your feet flat on the floor and your arms at your sides. Place your hands on the weights at chest height and face ahead while you lift.

2. Extend your arms completely aloft.

3. Put your hands back in the original position.

4. Do this ten times or as often as you feel necessary. Bicep curls, an excellent exercise for arm strength, may be performed almost anywhere.

Bicep Curls

This is a crucial biceps-building workout that requires dumbbells. Your biceps are constantly put to exercise as you lift, reach, open, and carry objects around. To avoid back discomfort, you should practice this exercise while seated in a chair. If your elbow hurts, you shouldn't do this exercise.

1. Hold the dumbbell in one hand down near your side while seated in a chair with your feet flat on the floor. Maintain an upright posture with your shoulders back and your palm facing inward.

2. Raise the load up toward your shoulder as you turn your hand upward.

3. Bring the load back to its original resting place.

4. Do this ten times or as often as you feel necessary.

5. Repeat with the other arm.

Triceps Extension

As with the previous arm workout, this one also benefits from the use of dumbbells. The triceps are a collection of muscles near the back of the upper arm that aid in shoulder and elbow motion. Stability and mobility in these areas, as well as overall mobility, will improve. Try this out while seated to avoid any unnecessary back strain. If your elbow hurts, you shouldn't do this exercise.

1. Place your feet flat on the ground, hip-width apart, and sit in a chair with a straight back. Raise the dumbbell, holding the right hand behind the head, close to the ear. Your left hand should be resting on your right elbow.

2. Raise your right arm straight up with your hand pointed upward. Keep supporting your elbow at all times.

3. Go back to the starting position.

4. Do this ten times or as often as you feel necessary.

Front Shoulder Raises

Front raises with a dumbbell are another fantastic shoulder and back exercise. A medicine ball, resistance band, or dumbbells are all good options. I advise doing this exercise while seated in a chair to avoid injuring your lower back and shoulders. If you're experiencing any sort of elbow pain, you should definitely skip this workout.

1. Keep your back straight and your hips as far back as you can in the chair. Make sure your feet are flat on the floor, and your shoulders are relaxed.

2. Let your arms hang at your sides, dumbbells in hand, palms facing toward your body.

3. You can even out the resistance band's length by squeezing it under the seat or sitting on it to make sure it's the same

on both sides. Hang your arms to the side, holding one end of the band in each hand, palms facing toward your body.

4. The medicine ball should be placed on the knees while holding on to both ends.

5. Raise the weight until it is even with your shoulders, keeping your arms at a right angle to your body. They need to be flat on the ground. Keep your palms facing each other and do not turn them outward.

6. Return to the original position gradually.

7. Perform 10 times.

Bent-Over Rows

You can strengthen your back, shoulders, arms, and core with this dumbbell exercise. Don't practice this exercise if your back or elbows hurt. When performing bent-over rows, it is possible to prevent injury by maintaining proper posture. Maintain a neutral spine when performing this exercise.

1. Position yourself such that your right hand is resting on the back of a solid chair. Hinge at the hips while bending over, keeping the back straight, and take a step back from the chair. To begin, you'll want to get into a squatting position with a slight bend in your knees and a dumbbell in your left hand.

2. Raise the dumbbell until it is even with your shoulder by pulling it up while bending at the left elbow.

3. Return to the original position gradually.
4. Do this ten times or as often as you feel necessary.
5. To perform the exercise with the opposite arm, you need to switch the dumbbell to your right hand.

If you want to see results from your workout, it's best to combine cardio with weightlifting. Combat heart disease by getting some exercise and taking a stroll around the block. The exercise will help you get in shape, and you'll have fun while taking in the sights, sounds, and company of the world around you. If you want to maintain your active lifestyle for as long as possible, you need to move as much as possible. Similarly, yoga and tai chi are acceptable alternatives. Both will help you maintain your balance and range of motion, which will have a beneficial effect on your weight training. Even more than that, they encourage a state of mind similar to meditation, which will help you relax and unwind.

Even though I encourage physical activity, I also recommend that rest is good for your health. Always pay attention to what your body is telling you. If you are hurting or tired, rest. Take some time to relax and let your heart rate and blood pressure return to normal. Overtraining, which frequently results in damage, is a major issue in the fitness industry. Rather than giving up, keep trying. The effects will become apparent.

What Happens to Your Muscle Mass and Strength as You Get Older?

By the age of 30, muscle mass naturally begins to decline. After this point, it falls even further during retirement. It also causes a weakening of the muscles. Research found that over the course of 7 years, the grip strength of elderly males decreased by 20%. Muscle and strength decline with age, making it more difficult for seniors to engage in their favorite hobbies and combat other age-related health issues like falling.

Muscles lose some of their cross-sectional area and girth as we get older. Fewer muscle fibers remain, and those that do shrink in size. Due to this weakness and muscle atrophy, even routine movements like opening a jar become more challenging. Muscle wasting is a recognized symptom of aging. One of the most important issues of aging is sarcopenia, which causes a person to become less functional and less able to care for themselves.

Muscle mass and the total number of muscle fibers both decline with age, but the proportion of fat to lean body mass increases. Aging seems to affect the fast-twitch muscle fibers that create more force than the slow-twitch fibers that are used for aerobic and endurance training.

The good news is that strength training can help you avoid or perhaps reverse some of this loss of muscle mass and strength as you age. Muscles can continue to develop and strengthen as we age. According to studies, three months of strength training resulted in considerable increases in muscular cross-sectional area and strength for older men. No matter your age, you should be doing some sort of strength exercise.

Loss of muscle mass and strength are two of the many bad things that come with getting older, but they can be helped with the right diet. There is evidence to show that elderly people have a higher protein requirement. Elderly people, depending on their level of activity, may require as much as 1.5 grams per kilogram of body weight, up from the recommended 0.8 grams per kilogram. When people get older, they lose some of their capacity to absorb proteins.

One study found that older people who took supplements with omega-3 fatty acids also made more muscle protein than those who took supplements with maize oil. Wild salmon, which is high in omega-3s, is just one example of a fatty fish that can be part of a healthy diet that can help slow down the natural decline in muscle mass that occurs with getting older. Lack of vitamin D can lead to a loss of muscle strength and sarcopenia, which are real and serious health problems.

Strength Training Techniques for Elderly Adults

Strength training for older people can help them get fit, stay independent, and have fewer health problems related to age-related conditions like heart disease, diabetes, arthritis, osteoporosis, and obesity. The Centers for Disease Control and Prevention suggest 150 minutes a week of moderate endurance activity. Cardiovascular activity, weight training, and bodyweight activities can all be included in this category. What older people should know about the benefits of strength training and how to get started is outlined below.

Muscle strength declines at a rate of 2%–4% annually after age 50. Muscle mass decreases at the rate of 3% annually after age 60, which equates to around 4.5 pounds lost annually. Since exercise delays cell aging, strength training not only helps you restore lost muscle but also keeps your cells looking youthful. Exercise does more than just refresh your body and mind. It has the potential to halt the chromosomal aging process. By building and keeping muscle mass, you can stop the loss of mobility, depression, and mental decline that come with getting older. Strength training should be part of a healthy older adult's exercise program at least twice per week, and research suggests that doing so as often as three or four times per week is safe.

The beneficial and restorative effects of strength exercise are hard to overestimate. Smart strength exercise that is gentle on the joints is essential for those over the age of 50. If you're having trouble with your joints, this may help tremendously. Don't neglect full-range-of-motion exercises, as these help your muscles learn how to keep you in control of your body in action. We don't really need all those high-tech, plush-upholstered circuit machines that require the user to sit in one location while they press and pull on various levers and buttons. We need to stand up from our chairs and move around more. Move your feet in a variety of ways. Moving your whole body should not hurt, but it should be enjoyable.

If the idea of lifting weights scares you, start with bodyweight exercises to learn how to do them correctly and avoid injury. There are several methods for gaining muscle mass and strength, and lifting weights is just one of them. Someone who can't raise their own weight shouldn't be trusted with anything heavier. People tend to move too fast, compromising form and biomechanics in order to lift heavy loads. Get started with the following routines:

- Squats

- Lunges

- Push-ups (on your back, your knees, or your toes)

- Dips

- Shoulder presses (holding up water bottles or raising your hands)

- Step-ups

- Bicycle crunches (three times a week, do two or three sets of ten to fifteen repetitions)

These exercises can help you in your day-to-day life. You can make the workout harder by using dumbbells or resistance bands. On days that aren't dedicated solely to strength training, do cardio or walk to aid with recovery. These are the exercises I recommend to beginners because they strengthen the body's major muscle groups through activities that are useful in everyday life, such as walking up and down stairs, carrying heavy bags of groceries, and playing with grandchildren. The two workouts that experts recommend the most for seniors are squats and push-ups. Squats help you get up from low surfaces like a chair or couch by building muscle in your legs and trunk.

As people get older, their leg and buttock strength goes down, making it hard for them to move around. If you start to feel weak, simple tasks like getting out of bed will become more challenging. Thus, put in a lot of time perfecting your squats. Also, practice push-ups from a wide variety of positions. If you fall, a push-up is a must-do action. You can be stuck for a long time if you don't try to pull yourself up. If you have some upper-body strength, you can at least roll over and yell for assistance.

Along with strength training, older people should do exercises for balance, flexibility, and mobility (range of motion). Employ a method of working out that covers a wide range of issues. Do exercises that work all of your muscles at once instead of just one at a time. Your strength gains will last longer if you also work on making yourself more mobile and flexible. If you lose your balance, you are more likely to fall, which can cause serious injuries. Experts focus most of their attention on exercises that help older people improve their range of motion and stability. For instance, performing a reach while standing on one leg can help you exercise and correct any muscle imbalances by engaging the joints.

- Raise the foot of one knee up to the level of the ankle of the opposite leg.

- Raise your supporting leg and bend the knee just a little.

- Raise one leg and reach forth with your foot, taking your time.

- Put your raised leg down and resume your starting positions.

- After a set, you can switch legs and repeat.

There has never been a more important time to pay attention to your pre- and post-exercise routines. The body just needs more time to repair itself than it did even a few decades ago. Keep in mind that you need to schedule additional downtime between strength training sessions and rest days in general. The main differences between exercising in your 20s and in your 60s are recovery and flexibility. It is possible that you will need some time to get back into the swing of things if you are not accustomed to lifting weights or haven't done it since you were younger. First-time resistance trainees should keep their workouts light and simple on day one. 10–15 minutes should be your target. If you're still feeling sore the next day, take a rest day. If you want to get the most out of your workouts, you must give your body time to adjust and recover after each session.

Big ambitions, like trying to lift a certain amount of weight, can be enticing. But it is more beneficial to determine the motivation behind your desire to maintain your strength and fitness. Think about what you want out of life now and what you need. Why do we bother with training if it doesn't seem to accomplish anything? The end result should inform the design of the strength and conditioning regimen. The potential for long-term sickness is also a major factor. As you age, your vulnerability to disease and other health issues increases. This may hinder your training. Yoga and Tai Chi are excellent additions to a healthy lifestyle because they improve mental health and help you relax. One of the most important aspects of aging with strength is the ability to move around freely and enthusiastically, even as one gets older.

Chapter 5

Nourishment for Optimal Regeneration

A Guide to Nutrition for Endurance Athletes

If you're new to triathlon, cycling, or running, you might feel overwhelmed when you see your training partners wearing what looks like a utility belt full of different kinds of food. This chapter is a resource for people who want to know more about the things that have been shown to help people stay energetic and perform at their best during endurance training and competition.

Carbohydrates 101

Sugars and starches are carbs, and they serve the same purpose for our bodies as gasoline does for a race vehicle. There are four calories of energy in every gram of carbohydrates. Humans, like race cars, store excess carbohydrates as glycogen in their muscle tissue and liver. Our bodies rely on these glycogen stores to maintain steady blood sugar levels and efficient muscular activity. Runners can meet their daily energy needs by storing glycogen in their muscles at a rate of about 2 grams (8 calories) and in their liver at a rate of about 100–125 grams (400–500 calories), assuming that 45–65% of their diet is made up of carbohydrates. Carbohydrate supplements are needed to avoid depletion, which can cause dizziness (called "bonking") and a lot of muscle fatigue (called "hitting the wall") during long runs. This is because the energy this amount of glycogen provides is only adequate for a moderately brisk two-hour run.

How much carbohydrate intake is required by athletes?

Race Week: If you're going to be competing in a race lasting more than three hours, you should "load" your body with carbs by eating four to five grams of simple (low fiber) carbohydrate content on a per-pound basis of lean body mass every day in the final 72 hours before the event. Carbohydrate loading is a term used to describe this method. Short-term carbo-loading programs that last only one or two days may be beneficial if the athlete continues to exercise up until the race and does not reduce training before the event. Pretzels, white pasta, white rice, plain bagels, bananas, potatoes, rice-based cereals, energy bars, and sports drinks are all examples of foods that are high in carbohydrates but are easy to digest.

Race Morning: Eat 100–150 grams of simple (low-fiber) carbs two to three hours before the start of the race. Make sure you give your body at least an hour to process every 200–300 calories you eat. A simple bagel spread with peanut butter and honey, along with 20 to 24 ounces of sports drink, is a good example of a pre-race breakfast that should be had between two and three hours before the start of the race.

During Race: After 45–90 minutes of exercise or competition, you should consume about a quarter to a third of your body weight in grams each hour. For every hour of running, a person of average weight (180 lbs) should eat 45–60 grams of carbohydrates. It has been shown that choosing foods with a long list of carbohydrate types increases the amount of glucose that your muscles can use, which makes you stronger. Maltodextrin, glucose, dextrose, sucrose, and fructose are all carbohydrate sources that are often used in sports nutrition products. Sports beverages, gels, bars, and chews are all common choices for pre- and post-race nutrition.

Post-Race: Get between 50 and 100 grams of carbs as soon as possible after a hard training session or race, preferably in the form of a liquid that will help you rehydrate and replenish your glucose.

Protein 101

About twenty percent of our total weight is made up of various tissues and body fluids, as well as other huge, complicated molecules. They include muscle, bone, cartilage, skin, and more. Amino acids are made when protein is broken down, and they are used to make many things, like skin, hair, nails, eyes, muscles, enzymes, antibodies, hormones, and chemicals in nerve cells. Research suggests that eating a small amount of protein while working out for a long time can improve performance by keeping glycogen in the muscles and making it easier to take in fluids. When working for longer periods of time, protein can help suppress hunger. However, excessive amounts of protein can cause a "backlog" of nutrients in the intestines, leading to gastrointestinal irritation and muscular fatigue or cramping if consumed too quickly after eating.

How much protein should an athlete consume?

In Training: Protein intake recommendations for endurance athletes range from 0.45 to 0.75 grams per pound of lean body mass per day. Targeting the upper end of this advice is ideal for athletes on low-calorie diets. A man who weighs 180 pounds but has only 10 percent body fat needs between 80 and 120 grams of protein per day because his lean body mass is 160 pounds.

Race Morning: In the two to three hours before the race, eat 10–20 grams of protein to keep your blood sugar level steady. Peanut butter, nonfat milk or yogurt, eggs, and energy bars are all good options for a pre-race protein snack.

During Race: Aim for up to 5 grams of protein every hour if you plan on being out on the course for longer than 4 hours for training or racing. Sports drinks and energy bars are popular options, but nutritious foods like turkey jerky and peanut butter sandwiches are also good sources.

Post-Race: It's enough to eat 10–20 grams of protein in the first hour after a race to help repair muscles and boost the immune system. Milk, meal replacement shakes, and sports drinks designed for recovery are all common examples.

Electrolytes 101

Electrolytes need to be replaced after endurance efforts that last longer than an hour, especially when training or competing in hot and humid conditions. Sodium is one of the main electrolytes, along with potassium, magnesium, and calcium. It is usually mixed with chloride. Electrolytes are important for the proper functioning of all cells, including muscles, because they are used in metabolic processes. Symptoms of an electrolyte imbalance include dehydration, nausea, vomiting, muscle weakness, muscle cramps, twitching, general weariness, hard breathing, "pins and needles," and confusion.

How many electrolytes are required for athletes to perform optimally?

Pre-Race: Athletes who compete in hot weather or who get muscle cramps and get tired easily may benefit from taking in more salt in the days before the competition. Pretzels, sports drinks, breads, and cereals are just some of the carbo-loading possibilities that can be adjusted for this. Also, on race day, it could be beneficial to consume a salt bagel, or sports drink instead of plain water and other low-salt foods like fruit and yogurt. Those who are taking blood pressure medication should not engage in salt loading.

During the Race: Aim for 200–500 mg of salt in every regular-cycle bottle of water (20–24 ounces). This is in addition to smaller amounts of magnesium, potassium, and calcium. Keep in mind that consuming too much sodium can cause gas and gastrointestinal distress, so keep track of how much sodium you take in from all sources.

Including:

- Shews [20-210 mg per 3 pieces]

- Sports drinks [100-200 mg per 8 oz]

- Electrolyte capsules [100-200 mg per capsule])

- Salt packets [200 mg per packet]
- Energy gels [25-200 mg per packet]

Post-Race: The best way to rehydrate your muscles after a race is with a sports drink, which also contains the electrolytes that your body lost.

Water 101

If you don't drink enough water before, during, and after a long run, you could seriously compromise your health and performance in the long run by dehydrating your body. Water is necessary for life because it is the medium for all metabolic processes, it cushions our muscles and joints, and it keeps our body temperature stable. Hence, it is crucial for athletes to know how much fluid they need to replace sweat. When training or competing, losing more than 2% of your body weight through sweat is unhealthy. You can avoid this by checking your weight before and after workouts and drinking enough water.

What is the recommended water intake for athletes?

Daily: Get half your weight in fluid ounces in order to have pale yellow pee throughout the day. For instance, a man who weighs 150 pounds needs to drink about 75 ounces of liquid per day.

Pre-Race: As 1-2% of your body's water weight is lost overnight, many people find it convenient to check their weight first thing in the morning. To avoid the bad effects of dehydration on performance, drink 16 to 24 ounces of fluid an hour or two before the race starts, or until your urine is pale yellow.

During-Race: In order to keep your urine from turning dark yellow, you should drink about 12 to 1 liter, or 1 normal bike bottle (20 to 24 ounces), per hour. Overhydration happens when you drink more water or other fluids than your body can absorb. This is also called hyponatremia. Clear urine, nausea, vomiting, pressure headaches, and confusion are some of the hallmarks of overhydration. Weighing yourself before and after an exercise is a good way to check how well you're hydrating. Aim for a weight loss of no more than 2 percent from your starting point.

Post-Race: If you sweated so much during your workout or race that you lost more than 2% of your pre-exercise weight, you need to replenish those fluids so that your urine is once again a pale yellow. For every pound of body weight that needs to be replaced, the standard suggestion is to consume 20 ounces of fluid.

Caffeine, the Bonus Ingredient

Caffeine's ability as a central nervous system stimulant to lessen tiredness, effort, discomfort, and pain in working muscles and the nervous system suggests that it may be useful for keeping blood glucose levels stable and stopping power loss.

The recommended caffeine intake for athletes

Two to three hours before the race, consume 100 to 300 milligrams of caffeine (e.g., one to three cups of coffee), and then take an additional 25 to 50 milligrams of caffeine hourly or add them near the end of the race. On the day of the race, don't take in more than 500 milligrams of caffeine. The best outcomes can be achieved by avoiding caffeine for at least 10 days before the race.

Everything You Need to Know About the Ideal Diet for Fitness Training

Proper fitness nutrition

Even more than physical setbacks, bad eating habits are the main reason why training fails too soon. A diet full of nutrients should be at the center of any plan to get stronger and fitter. Advice on what to eat can help you provide your body with the pure fuel it needs to thrive.

How to Improve Your Diet: Suggestions and Recommendations

Keep a food diary: Keeping a food journal can assist you in keeping tabs on not just what you eat but also how much, when, and where you eat it. Try keeping a food and mood journal for a single day. Put an end to all cheating! Calculate the total number of calories for the following day. There's a chance that you won't be happy with your calorie intake. Your intake of protein, carbohydrates, and fats, as well as your progress toward meeting the Recommended Daily Allowance (RDA) for numerous essential vitamins and minerals, may all be calculated by using one of the many available free online trackers or apps. Not only what you eat, but also when you eat it, should be recorded. Some people keep diaries detailing their eating habits and the people they were with at the time to determine if they were motivated to overeat due to their emotions.

Calculate calories: Most diets tell you to eat a certain number of calories per day, like 1,500 or 2,000 for people who are moderately active. There are a plethora of free applications and websites that can tell you how many calories you need to eat to maintain your weight, how many calories you need to eat to lose weight, and everything in between. For instance, www.calculator.net has tools like body mass index calculators and calorie counters. Use these to determine your daily calorie and nutritional requirements. The results of your food diary and the calculator can provide some eye-opening comparisons. www.myfitnesspal.com is another helpful tool for monitoring calorie consumption. Download this free app onto your mobile device and gain access to the largest nutrition and calorie database in the world, which now has information on more than 5 million distinct items. You can easily keep tabs on the calories you consume while on the road!

Weigh and measure your food: That may be annoying to measure at first, but you'll quickly adapt. It will also help you realize which foods are worth the calories and which are unnecessary fillers. You can use this information to make healthier food decisions. It would be worthwhile to get a food scale—a miniature scale capable of measuring weight in ounces and grams. Having a basic set of measuring implements, such as cups and spoons, might also be useful for this purpose. Using a measuring cup to pour a predetermined amount into a preferred cup or bowl is a simple approach to establishing portion control. One cup, half a cup, etc., will have a much more concrete visual representation for you when you observe how much actually fits into your preferred bowl.

Eat the right food: For optimal performance in sports and weight training, a diet low in processed foods is recommended. If you want to reduce weight, lean protein, complex carbohydrates, and fiber can help you immensely. Protein helps your body in several ways, including muscular growth, weight maintenance, and satiety. In addition to providing you with sustained energy, complex carbohydrates like those found in green, leafy vegetables also help to keep your digestive system and hormones functioning normally. Monounsaturated fats like olive oil or plant-based sources high in omega-3 fatty acids should be used for fat consumption. Omega-3 fatty acids can be found in walnuts, flaxseed oil, and other related nuts and seeds.

Don't eat the wrong foods: Unless you carefully read the labels, you should avoid eating from boxes or bags. Added sugar, salt, and preservatives are common in processed foods. Ignore the marketing and start comparing labels instead. The use of deceptive marketing terms, such as "natural" and "healthy," on food packaging can be a major contributor to weight gain and cardiovascular problems. While reading the label on a product, you should always start at the top to find the ingredients that have the highest concentration. If you must eat packaged goods, prioritize those with labels that sound like "real food" and avoid those with unpronounceable chemical names. Save processed foods for special occasions or as a last resort.

Limit your drinking: Calories can quickly add up when you drink alcohol. Drinking alcohol can quickly add 400–500 calories to your daily intake, and much more if you enjoy mixing your liquor with sugary mixes. Alcohol is metabolized for fuel before any other kind of fuel in the body, leading some nutritionists to conclude that the calories you take from alcoholic beverages are the worst kind of calories you can consume. It's possible that the food you eat will be turned into fat at a much higher rate if you're also drinking. A serious athlete should avoid alcohol. Its drawbacks are greater than its advantages.

Drink water: To put it simply, water is the best thirst reliever in the natural world. Have plenty of clean water every day, and have some with every meal. Take in 16 ounces, or two cups, of water around two hours before hitting the gym. Keep hydrating with water as you work out. Drink more water than you think you need if you plan on working out in hot weather. Indicative of mild dehydration, thirst prompts you to replenish fluid stores. Keep hydrated to stave off thirst.

Avoid sugar: Fructose in fruits and other natural sweeteners like maple syrup and honey are just a few examples. Refined white sugar is a poor source of nutrition, serving primarily as fuel. It's been linked to dental decay and weight gain. Try eating something sweet like fruit for dessert instead of adding sugar to your diet.

Weight Lifting Nutrition

Nutritional protein sources that are particularly useful for weight training include the following:

- **Egg protein**: Bodybuilders and weightlifters used to mix raw eggs into a glass of milk to make their protein shakes. Salmonella infection fears have made the consumption of raw eggs taboo nowadays. Eggs that have been properly cooked are edible. In contrast to the yolks (the yellow part in the middle), which are high in fat and cholesterol, egg whites are a lean source of protein. The biological value (BV) of egg protein is 100.

- **Meat**: Protein-rich beef, pork, and chicken all have a B.V. of 80. Leaner cuts, especially when baked rather than fried, are a rich source of protein in the diet despite the fact that they might be high in fat. Including fish in your protein-rich diet is a viable option.

- **Plants**: There are vegetarian weightlifters who are quite powerful and fit, and they acquire all of the protein they require from plant sources rather than animal products. Protein can be found in vegetables, but only in a fraction of the amounts seen in animal products. The combination of beans and nutritious grains like rice or quinoa is a great way to get a lot of protein in one meal. Protein-rich but also fat-rich, nuts and seeds are a healthy addition to any diet. Raw nuts and seeds are preferable to roasted versions because of the extra salt and fat that can be added during the roasting process.

Meal Frequency and Timing

Athletes should eat many small meals throughout the day to keep their bodies in the best shape possible. By eating every two to three hours, you can keep your energy up and get the most out of the nutrients that help you build muscle. If you're going to eat, don't just eat carbs. When eating a high-carb meal, it's best to pair it with protein or fat to reduce the insulin spike. After eating, you may feel even more famished due to the subsequent crash. If you feel hungry between meals, reach for a protein-rich snack. When it comes to muscle repair and growth after exercise, nothing beats a protein-rich diet. Get hydrated well before hitting the gym.

Bringing It All Together: A Course of Action for You

The best method to stay in shape is to combine proper nutrition with some sort of personal exercise program. The first step toward success is figuring out what foods you need and how much of them you need to eat. To be in great shape, you have to find the right balance of protein, fat, and carbohydrates in your diet. Possible components of your strategy are:

- Keeping a food journal or using a food tracking website or app to keep track of what you eat, how much, and when

- Determining the appropriate calorie intake for weight maintenance, weight gain, or weight loss

- By measuring and weighing your food, you can control how much you consume at each meal.

- Preferring whole, unprocessed foods instead of processed ones.

- Reducing your use of sugary juices, sodas (including diet sodas), and alcoholic beverages and increasing your water intake is a good place to start.

- Consume protein-rich foods like lean meats or eggs after weight training sessions to speed up muscle healing and growth.

- Monitoring your state of health after implementing dietary adjustments. These aren't temporary adjustments made in preparation for a single competition. Until they make you feel good, you won't be sticking with them.

- Keeping tabs on how far you've come. How effective have the adjustments been thus far? If not, what dietary adjustments can you make to get there?

Weightlifters and serious athletes of all kinds rely heavily on protein. Keep in mind that your body is a temple and that the food you eat is like the bricks that make up the walls. Avoid highly processed foods if you want to achieve a lean, muscular physique. Eat the highest-quality meals you can afford, take a protein supplement, and drink plenty of clean water. Stay away from salt, sugar, and alcohol. Support your body's transformation toward your ideal fitness level by giving it what it needs to get there: plenty of rest and outdoor exercise.

Fats You Should (and Shouldn't) Eat While Training

Here are the fats you should eat and the ones you should stay away from while training to keep your performance and body composition at their best.

Training Nutrition: Which Fats Are Best?

Nuts

Healthy fats can be found in nuts like almonds, pistachios, walnuts, and peanuts. Nuts are a good source of unsaturated fat, which has been shown to lower inflammation and speed up healing. Also, eating nuts has been linked to a reduced threat of cardiovascular disease. Before hitting the gym, a tablespoon of nut butter can be a good idea. Combine walnuts with Greek yogurt for a post-workout snack; The omega-3 fatty acids found in walnuts have anti-inflammatory effects.

Seeds

Smoothies, salads, and energy balls can all benefit from the addition of chia, flax, and hemp seeds, which are rich in omega-3s. Even though they don't contribute much flavor, they are a welcome source of extra protein and texture. You may also bread other meats like chicken, fish, and steak with them to achieve a satisfying crunchy exterior. Since seeds reduce inflammation, you may be able to train harder, heal faster, and feel less pain in your muscles if you eat them.

Avocado

Avocados are different from other fruits because they have monounsaturated fats, which help reduce inflammation, are good for your heart, and make you feel full. Avocados have 20 different vitamins and minerals, plus potassium and important phytonutrients. This makes them great foods to eat after a workout to help your body recover.

Olive Oil

This oil is part of the Mediterranean diet because it is high in heart-healthy unsaturated fats. Pour it over grilled vegetables or a salad.

Salmon

It's advised that you eat fish at least twice a week, and one of those times should be salmon. It has a high concentration of omega-3 fatty acids, which are good for your heart, and the fat makes you feel full, so you don't crave sweets after dinner. Also, the vitamin D in salmon helps strengthen bones and keep people from getting hurt.

Avoid these fatty foods while working out.

Bacon

Bacon has a lot of saturated fat, salt, and nitrates, all of which are linked to a higher risk of heart disease as well as fluid retention, dehydration, gas, and bloating. Try to find a brand that doesn't include nitrates or nitrites, and if you must eat it, swap it out with lean turkey sausage or grilled chicken.

Packaged Desserts

Oftentimes, packaged desserts contain not only the sugar we'd expect to find but also trans-fat, which is so dangerous that many restaurants have banned its use. Read the label carefully and stay away from anything that says "partially hydrogenated oil," which is a trans-fat.

Butter

Saturated fats are found primarily in butter. Too much butter in the diet is dangerous for the cardiovascular system. The percentage of calories from saturated fat in your diet should not exceed 5%. That's 11 grams of saturated fat for a 2,000-calorie diet. Butter comprises 7 grams of saturated fat per tablespoon, so use only a small amount if you must have it in your meal.

The Role of Nutrition in Muscle Growth

If you want to bulk up, you need to pay equal attention to what you eat and how much exercise you get. Although pushing your body physically is important, your progress will stall if you don't also provide it with the nutrients it needs. Protein-rich foods are important for building muscle, but carbs and lipids are also needed. Gaining lean muscle requires a commitment to regular exercise and an increase in caloric intake from muscle-building sources.

Foods that help you gain muscle and get lean

Eggs

Eggs are a great source of protein, healthy fats, and other nutrients like B vitamins and choline, all of which are necessary for building muscle and keeping one's energy levels up.

Salmon

Salmon is a great food for building muscle and staying healthy because it is high in protein (17 grams per serving), omega-3 fatty acids (1.5 grams per serving), and healthy B vitamins. Omega-3 fatty acids can help your muscles grow and recover when you eat them before, during, and after your workouts.

Chicken breast

In a 3-ounce serving, chicken breasts have 26.7 grams of high-quality protein. This makes them a great source of protein for building muscle. They also have the B vitamins niacin and b6 that help the body work normally while exercising. It has been shown that diets high in protein, such as those that include chicken, aid weight loss.

Greek yogurt

Dairy is a great source of protein since it contains both fast- and slow-digesting types (casein and whey). Studies have shown that eating these proteins together leads to greater gains in lean body mass. But not all dairy products are the same; Greek yogurt, for example, typically has twice as much protein as regular yogurt. Greek yogurt is a healthy snack, but it may be especially useful after working out or before bed.

Tuna

Vitamins A and B, which are both found in tuna in large amounts, are important for good health, lots of energy, and top physical performance. It's rich in omega-3 fatty acids, which may help keep muscles healthy and prevent the natural decline in strength and size that comes with getting older.

Lean beef

Beef is a healthy choice because it has protein, B vitamins, minerals, and the amino acid creatine. Eating lean red meat has been shown to help people gain lean muscle mass when they lift weights. Lean beef is great for building muscle because it helps stimulate muscle growth without adding too many calories.

Shrimp

Protein-rich shrimp are convenient and healthy because they are low in fat and calories yet high in muscle-building protein. The nutritional breakdown per 3-ounce portion is as follows: 19 g of protein, 1.44 g of fat, and 1 g of carbohydrates. Leucine, an amino acid essential for proper muscle development, is also abundant in shrimp.

Soybeans

Half a cup of cooked soybeans is packed with nutrients, including protein (16 grams), healthy unsaturated fats (8 grams), and vitamins and minerals like vitamin K, iron, and phosphorus (all 3 grams).

Cottage cheese

Low-fat cottage cheese has 28 grams of protein and the amino acid leucine, which helps build muscle. It comes in low-fat, medium-fat, and high-fat forms, with the high-fat from having the most calories. Whether you go for low-fat or full-fat cottage cheese depends on how many calories you're looking to add to your diet.

Turkey breast

Turkey breast has about 26 grams of protein per 3-ounce (85-gram) meal and nearly no fat or carbohydrates. Turkey has a lot of niacin, a B vitamin that is needed to break down fats and carbohydrates. Building muscle takes time and effort, but if your B vitamin levels are appropriate, your body will respond positively to training, and you'll see results faster.

Tilapia

Tilapia is a seafood option that is high in protein. It has 23 grams of protein and is also a good source of vitamin B12 and selenium. You can't bulk up without vitamin B12, which helps your nerves and blood cells function properly.

Beans

Beans are high in plant-based protein, magnesium, phosphorus, fiber, B vitamins, and iron, all of which have been linked to long-term health benefits and preventing disease. Beans like black, pinto, and kidney beans, as well as other common types, have about 15 grams of protein and a lot of fiber and B vitamins per cup.

Protein powders

Even though whole foods are the foundation of a healthy diet, supplements can sometimes help. Supplementing your diet with protein shakes is a good idea if you have problems consuming enough protein through food alone. Most people choose dairy-based protein powders like whey and casein. Some of these powders use protein derived from plants like soy and peas or from animals like cows and chickens.

Edamame

Edamame, a form of immature soybean, offers 18 grams of protein and 8 grams of fiber per 100 grams. High levels of folate, vitamin K, and manganese help the body use amino acids, which may be important for keeping lean muscle mass and strength as you age.

Quinoa

One cup of cooked quinoa has forty grams of carbohydrates, eight grams of protein, five grams of fiber, and significant levels of magnesium and phosphorus. The muscles and nerves you use to move around require magnesium to operate properly.

Scallops

Scallops are high in protein and low in fat, just like shrimp, tilapia, and chicken. These very lean protein sources may be great if you're trying to increase your protein intake without dramatically increasing your calorie intake. About 17 grams of protein and less than 100 calories can be found in three ounces (85 grams) of scallops.

Lean jerky

On the go, you may have a craving for lean jerky or another high-protein meat snack. Because jerky may be manufactured from a wide variety of meats, its nutritional value will change depending on the type of meat used. While the majority of the fat is removed during processing, the protein still accounts for the majority of the snack's calorie value. These types of animal proteins are of higher quality and aid in muscle growth.

Chickpeas

Chickpeas, or garbanzo beans, have a lot of both carbohydrates and protein. There are about 15 grams of protein, 45 grams of carbohydrates, and 13 grams of fiber in a 1-cup (164-gram) portion of canned chickpeas.

Peanuts

With 7 grams of protein, 6 grams of carbohydrates, and a lot of healthy unsaturated fat, peanuts are a fantastic multi-nutrient source. Peanuts have about 166 calories per serving size of 1 ounce and have more of the amino acid leucine than other plant foods.

Buckwheat

A lot of people consume buckwheat since it's high in magnesium, manganese, B vitamins, and phosphorus, all of which are good for you and may be used to keep you healthy and even build muscle.

Tofu

Tofu, made from soy milk, is a popular vegetarian alternative to traditional meat dishes. There are 10 grams of protein, 6 grams of fat, and 2 grams of carbs in a half-cup portion of raw tofu (124 grams). Calcium, which is found in tofu, is good for your bones and muscles. Good sources of plant-based protein include soy products like tofu. Vegans and vegetarians can benefit from eating foods made with soy protein.

Pork tenderloin

Tenderloin provides 23.1 grams of protein per 4 ounces (113 grams) and only 2 grams of fat, making it a fantastically nutritious choice. Several studies have shown that pork is just as effective at building muscle as beef or chicken.

Milk

Milk is a complete source of nutrients because it contains protein, carbs, and lipids. Milk, like other dairy products, has proteins that are both quickly and slowly digested. For muscular development, this may be a good thing. Regular milk consumption and weight training can both help with muscle growth.

Almonds

Almonds have 6 grams of protein, magnesium, and phosphorus (vitamin E), and they help the body use carbs and fats as energy. Almonds should be eaten in moderation because of their high calorie content. More than 400 calories can be found in only a half cup of blanched almonds.

Bison

Bison has a similar amount of protein to beef (3 ounces = 85 grams) per serving. While beef has been shown to increase the risk of heart disease, bison may be a healthier option. Bison is a great alternative to beef if you're watching your weight and looking to add muscle mass without sacrificing flavor.

Brown rice

Brown rice has both the protein (6 grams per cup) and carbs (which give you energy during exercise) that you need to perform at your best. You may be able to exercise more intensely if you consume healthy food sources like brown rice or quinoa in the hours before you work out. Studies suggest that taking rice protein supplements during weight training can lead to just as much muscle growth as doing so with whey protein alone.

Preparing Balanced Meals for the Elderly

A diet full of healthy foods and regular physical activity can help us stay in good health as we age. Check out the links below to learn more about healthy eating habits and how to create a well-balanced diet. A better diet can be established with relatively minor changes. In order to maximize your dietary intake and achieve your nutrient needs while lowering your disease risk, consider the following:

- Reduce your chances of developing chronic diseases, including hypertension, heart disease, and diabetes, by eating a balanced diet that includes foods from all food groups. Choose foods that are low in saturated fat, added sugar, and sodium.

- To get enough protein and keep your muscles healthy, eat fish, dairy, fortified soy products, and legumes like beans, peas, and lentils every day.

- Make sure to include fresh fruits and vegetables, sliced or chopped, in all of your meals and snacks. Look for pre-cut alternatives if you have trouble slicing and chopping.

- Vitamin B12 can be found in some breakfast cereals and other foods; if you're not getting enough, talk to your doctor about getting a supplement. Take the time to educate yourself about essential nutrients.

- Herbs and citrus juices, including lemon juice, are great alternatives to salt that can be used to season cuisine.

- Drinking water often is a must if you want your digestion and absorption of nutrients to be better and if you want to stay hydrated all day. Put down the sugary drinks.

Making healthy eating choices and sticking with them might be challenging for some people..

USDA Food Patterns

As people age, their eating patterns often shift. The United States Department of Agriculture (USDA) created Food Patterns to explain several healthy diet options. Included in these dietary routines are:

- The U.S. Dietary Pattern (based on typical American food consumption) is a healthy way to eat. Whole grains,

- vegetables, fruits, seafood, poultry, and meat; fat-free or low-fat dairy products; as well as eggs, nuts, seeds, and soy products are the mainstays of this diet.

- The healthy Mediterranean diet includes more vegetables, fruits, and fish and less meat and dairy than the healthy American diet.

- A healthy vegetarian eating pattern is one that excludes all forms of meat, poultry, and fish while including fat-free or low-fat dairy products. More soy products, nuts and seeds, beans and peas, eggs, and whole grains can be found in this eating pattern than in the healthy U.S.-style eating pattern.

Meal planning

Prepare delicious and nutritious meals by following these guidelines:

- **Plan in advance.** If you have a plan, it's easier to get rid of hunger pangs and eat healthy food.

- **Find budget-friendly foods.** Make a list of what you need to buy in advance to help you save money.

- **Consider preparation time.** Five minutes is all you need to prepare some meals. If you enjoy cooking or are making dinner for a group of people, you might like to test your skills with a more complicated dish.

- **Keep calories in mind.** Calorie requirements change from person to person. Before making any drastic changes to your diet or exercise routine, be sure to consult with your doctor.

Recipes

Trying to find tasty-sounding recipes online might be an excellent starting point when it comes to dinner preparation. The USDA's **MyPlate Kitchen** is a great place to get nutritious meal ideas and make a shopping list. Based on your age, height, weight, and degree of physical activity. The **MyPlate Plan** tool will recommend a specific menu for you to follow.

Chapter 6

Mind-Muscle Connection and Mental Toughness

Acknowledging the Role of Mental Focus in Physical Performance

Aging brings about physical and mental changes. There's a chance they'll weaken, but there's also a chance they'll strengthen. Consider the brain: Keeping those synapses in check requires constant use in the form of learning and hard activities like solving puzzles. Then there are your muscular groups. Constantly tuning and pushing one's strength and fitness as one ages can help prevent the long-term effects of things like falls and other accidents.

But how does your mind change as you age? The more you focus on improving your physical strength, the more aware you'll become of the state of your entire body, and the more you'll be able to push yourself physically and mentally. If you don't understand how, you could accomplish it, then these tips should help.

Mind muscle connection tips

Turn off distractions

- Put away all distractions, like the TV or podcasts, and focus completely on your exercise routine.

Visualize the muscles you are training

- Focus on the muscle you are targeting with each rep. If you want to target a certain muscle group, you should bring your thoughts and energy to that spot.

Include warm-up sets

- Do a warm-up set of high reps with a light weight before attempting your actual lift. Focus on contracting the muscle you're trying to work by squeezing the weight.

Add cues

- It's possible to use either mental or external cues, such as instructing yourself to push your heels into the ground or rowing your elbows behind your body when performing a bench press.

Increase time under tension

The duration of each repetition is measured in terms of time under strain. For optimal brain-muscle-fiber communication, perform sets at a slower pace. If you want to build muscle faster, try tempo reps, in which you hold your muscular tension for two to three seconds at a time.

Uncovering the link between thought and action

The mind-muscle link can be defined as the intentional contraction of a muscle. The capacity to isolate a muscle or muscle group during exercise is the key difference between using light weights at random and getting a good workout. When you focus on contracting a certain muscle, the brain sends more fast-twitch muscle fibers to that muscle. As a consequence, this inhibits the innervation of resting muscle fibers. Focusing tension where it will do the best is essential for building muscle and mass where it matters most.

Paying close attention, both internally and externally

A high level of focused attention is the result of the brain's ability to pay close attention to one task for a prolonged period of time. This is not only a great tool for lifting weights, but it also helps your mind grow in important ways. When you're out and about, it's crucial to pay attention to both your body and your surroundings. Concentrating inward means giving one's full attention to one's physical actions. For instance, when performing a crunch, you may train your mind to concentrate on tightening the anterior abdominal muscles and flexing the spine.

How your body interacts with its surroundings during a workout constitutes an external focus. For instance, the exterior aim of a leg press machine is to move the platform away from the user's midsection. While both exterior and internal focus have been shown to boost performance, research suggests that internal focus is more crucial to the process of building muscle. Concentrate your thoughts and willpower on the muscles that will be doing the work. Consider how your biceps contract as you perform a biceps curl, bringing the weight up near your shoulder. Everything you do to build muscle should follow this rule.

Choosing one cue at a time

Cueing is a way for coaches and trainers to improve the performance and movement of their athletes. On your own time, you can use cueing to train your brain to communicate with the muscles. Check your form and make a note of the areas you want to improve. As soon as you have a few ideas for cues, focus on just one at a time. Here's an example: the bench press. You've done everything necessary: set up, drop the bar, and press it. Correct setup is the primary indicator of improvement. Taking the bar safely off the rack involves setting it up on the bench with your body tight and braced, then taking it down. Give your full attention to these abilities before your brain can settle on the correct posture and alignment. Once you know how to do this, you can move on to easier challenges that require less mental and physical effort. Focus can be improved over time by breaking down difficult movements into smaller pieces that are easier to practice.

More time under tension

Muscle growth relies heavily on time under tension during resistance exercise. Muscles get stronger and bigger the longer they're under tension during a lift. There are numerous strategies one might employ to prolong the period of stress. One method is to halt the contraction at its apex. For the glutes, you can hold at the top of a bridge; for the biceps, at the top of a flexed curl; or at the bottom of a push-up. Extending the eccentric phase of the exercise more slowly is another option. Adding a 3-second eccentric movement helps strengthen the link between your brain and your muscles because your mind naturally shifts its focus to controlling the slowed-down action. If you want to lengthen the time your muscles are under tension and strengthen the connection between your nerves and muscles, isometric contractions are a great way to do both. The plank is a fantastic illustration of an isometric contraction. Some more examples include isometric chin-ups, loaded carries, and iso-hold squats.

Turn off distractions

The idea that people can perform two things at once extends beyond the common practice of patting one's head while caressing one's belly. You might think you'll be able to go through your workout more quickly if you ignore the discomfort involved in achieving your goals. But in reality, the reverse is correct. Putting away the phone and the TV helps the mind concentrate on the work at hand. Listening to music before a workout might help get your blood pumping and get you in the zone, but audiobooks and podcasts may be better left for the couch.

Putting it all together

As you exercise, your mind and body can communicate in many different ways. Focusing takes practice, so pick one thing at a time and hone it as you learn more about your body. For starters, it's essential to get rid of all potential interruptions if you're just getting into exercising. Eccentric contractions are the most basic method of gaining muscle quickly. Veterans in the gym should concentrate on concentric and isometric contractions and incorporate cues into their workout to maximize their muscle-building potential.

What is mental toughness?

The two aspects of my definition of mental toughness are:

- The state of mind that allows for optimal performance under pressure

- The ability to overcome obstacles and emerge victorious.

Actors, executives, teachers, and students all use the phrase "mental toughness". However, it is most often used in sports.

Common Myths

Myth #1: You can't teach mental toughness.

False: It can be taught.

Studies that span more than seven decades show that mental toughness is not innate and can be taught to athletes and people of all ages, levels of experience, and personality types.

Myth #2: Only people with mental illnesses should participate in mental training.

False: Almost everyone may gain from it.

Although mental training may sound similar to therapies used to treat people with mental illness, there is a key distinction to be made. People with typical intelligence can achieve great success when they put their minds to work. Well-being is independent of both being sick and recovering from it.

Myth #3: It takes far too long to master it.

False: Everyone can fit in their workouts by combining digital tools with traditional methods.

There are a lot of online tools available to train mental toughness.

Myth #4: Physical toughness equals mental toughness.

False. – There is a distinction between them. And you have to focus on both at once if you want to reach your full potential.

The body's toughness is important.

Even if an athlete is mentally tough, they might not be able to do well in their sport without the physical toughness they need. Most athletes at the top levels of their sport are very fit and good at what they do. Thus, what separates a winner from a runner-up is mental fortitude.

Who is this for?

Everyone who is willing to put in the effort can benefit from developing mental toughness. Everybody in any field, from athletes and coaches to businesspeople and artists, can benefit from developing mental toughness. Only people who are happy with subpar performance won't benefit from it. Stop right now if you think "good enough" will do. Read on if you want to be the best at what you do.

Are you mentally tough?

Would you say that you have the mental fortitude to realize your wildest ambitions? Rather, you should ask yourself, "Am I mentally tough enough... yet?" Mental strength is a skill that can be acquired through training. Not everyone is born with a perfect set of mental abilities. Mastering your mental abilities is essential to reaching your full potential in your chosen field. Developing proficiency in this area requires time and effort. Those who are in charge of a child's or a child's performance should keep this in mind as well. The resilience of one's mentor seeps into one's own mind. If you want to communicate effectively with your coach, parent, or mentor, you also need to focus on your own mental abilities. So, what are the most typical indications that a person's cognitive abilities could use some work?

Signals That Your Mental Capacity Could Use Some Work

- Having trouble keeping your cool during high-stakes contests or games

- Low confidence

- Angry outbursts

- Lack of determination or reluctance to persist

- Difficulty focusing

- Poor starts or finishes

- Inadequate encouragement from authority figures

- A sense of external pressure from a coach, parent, or another authority figure.

- Reputational weight causes high standards to be placed on performance.

- The standard of performance in competition is lower than in practice.

- The mindset of "winning is everything" (outcome-focused)

- Inability to recover quickly from setbacks

- Fear of the competition Worrying about what other people will think of you or failing at something

You are not alone if any of the above describe you.

Strategies for Building Mental Toughness

The research found that less than 1% of young athletes train their minds, even though top athletes like Michael Jordan have shown that having a strong mind is important for success.

Why is that?

Many report feeling at a loss. If so, you're in luck, because that's what this section is all about.

How to ensure you have the resilience you need to succeed

How Can I Develop Mental Toughness?

Have you ever pursued something with such zeal that you refused to give up regardless of how difficult the going became? This is the essence of mental fortitude. The key is to maintain a positive attitude and act with fortitude despite the daunting challenges you may face. A person with strong mental fortitude truly believes that "Where there's a will, there's a way." They never give up hope, confidence, or self-belief, and they keep going even when things are hard. They do this with urgency, determination, and focused effort. These people are relentless in the pursuit of their greatest aspirations and passions. Even though they seem to be up against insurmountable odds, they keep going and eventually succeed. Whether they succeed or fail, they will come out of it stronger and wiser.

A person who gives up easily when they make a mistake, are rejected, or receive negative feedback cannot become mentally tough. In a similar vein, you can't do it if you can't deal with feelings of worry, panic, frustration, stress, or fear. If you can't handle doubt, pain, and impatience, then it's highly unlikely that you will succeed. Considering this, you could say that most of us don't have the emotional strength to get through the biggest problems we face. Why? That's because a lot of us are easily hurt and take things way too personally.

It is possible that you are the type of person who quits when the going gets tough. You might want to improve your ability to bounce back quickly from setbacks and stay strong when things don't go your way. Why do some people seem to have natural mental fortitude while others have to work so hard to get anywhere? The reality is that mental toughness isn't innate. Rather, it's a skill we hone over time. It's earned the hard way through the trials and tribulations we face.

When I say that it doesn't matter what happens to us, I mean exactly that. More than anything else, it's how we interpret events and how we respond to them that determines the course of our lives. Toughness of mind is a matter of personal choice rather than innate ability. Your mental toughness is a function of the choices you make in the here and now and the routines you develop over time. Mental toughness varies widely depending on the context. No one has the same experience as you or me. Everyone has their own standards for what constitutes mental fortitude under specific conditions. For you, what exactly is the standard? So, let's find out. Ponder these:

- How do I define mental toughness for myself?

- How do I know when I've proven my mental toughness in a given circumstance?

- How can I show myself that I am strong and resilient psychologically? What norms and guidelines will I follow?

- How can I prove to myself that I am strong psychologically? That I am strong enough to face any challenge that life may present?

In order to convince yourself that you can handle life's toughest problems, you should establish criteria to measure your success. It also serves as a gauge for your reactions and development. On the other hand, if you can't answer these questions definitively right now, that's fine too. As you read on, you will no doubt have more questions answered, and new ideas sparked.

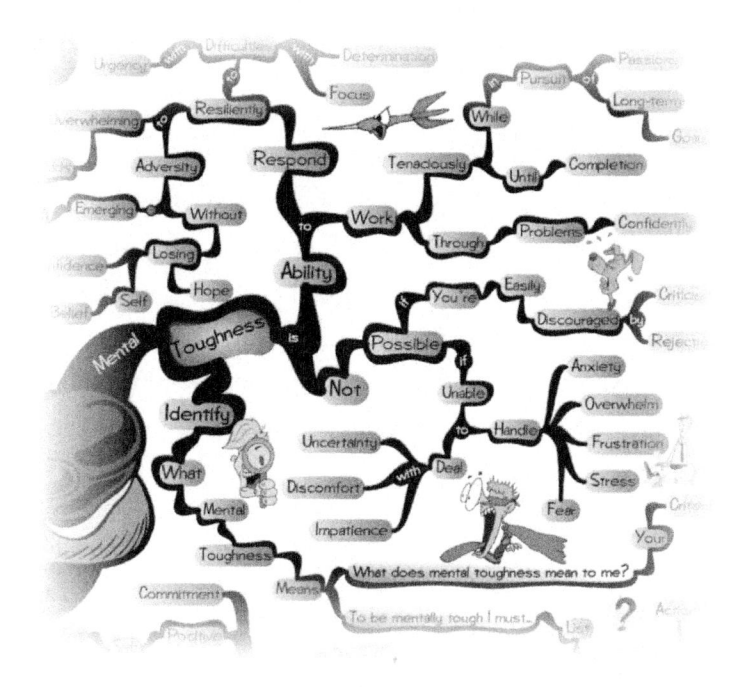

What You Need to Be Mentally Strong

How does one go about strengthening their resolve? Or, to put it another way, what are the necessary conditions for fostering this mental habit? To put it mildly, that's not a question with a simple solution. Develop your mental fortitude by actively working to improve your circumstances. Let's examine some of these in more detail.

You Need to Know What You're Trying to Achieve

To begin with, you must have objectives that will serve as a source of motivation. But these can't be generic, meaningless aspirations either. To be more effective, they should be driven by your deepest values and contribute to your life's greatest meaning. They should be the driving force behind every decision and action you take. They should have deep personal significance and inspire you to exert extra effort in their pursuit.

Determination and self-control are required.

Now that you have a plan in place, it's time to practice self-discipline to become mentally tough. Self-discipline is essential for maintaining concentration when external factors work against you. Also, you'll need a lot of inner fire to keep going in the face of adversity. And the first step in getting motivated is to talk to yourself in a way that is encouraging and upbeat.

You must give it your all.

Having mental fortitude also calls for a serious dedication to succeeding. When times are tough, you must be able to "stay the course" without wavering or hesitation. In order to succeed, you need to settle in for the long haul. You can overcome the obstacles you face by committing to making steady progress toward your goal.

You Must Feel a Calling and Take Responsibility

One way to be mentally tough is to go to work with a clear idea of your goals and responsibilities. It necessitates putting in effort for the greater good. There must be some greater purpose that motivates you every day. What this means is that you should have a good reason for doing whatever it is you plan on doing. In the absence of these things, one will lack the motivation to persevere through life's challenges.

You must be capable of handling pain.

To be mentally tough, one must be able to keep their feelings in check and not let them cloud their judgment. By doing this, you will be able to separate your feelings from the actual results of your efforts and focus on the steps you need to take to reach your goals. The same can be said for "mental toughness," which is the capacity to endure pain in the face of adversity. You need to train yourself to accept uncertainty as a part of life so that it doesn't cloud your ability to make sound judgments.

Maintain a practical perspective.

Maintaining a tough mentality involves knowing your limits and working within them. The key is, to be honest with yourself about your abilities, the resources at your disposal, and the amount of time you have available to complete the task. When things get tough, it's helpful to be able to make course corrections based on an honest assessment of the situation. Avoiding catastrophic blunders that could spell doom is a major benefit. Furthermore, it allows you to seek assistance before things spiral out of control.

Responsibility is something you must take very seriously.

Two-fold responsibility is needed for mental toughness. First and foremost, you have to be responsible for your own decisions and actions. If you say it, it must be done. Your word is law, and you will do everything in your power to make it happen. Consider: How will you ensure that you follow through? Secondly, you need to have other people hold you to your word. People who are responsible for holding you accountable will not put up with any nonsense from you. Because of the increased scrutiny that comes with increased accountability, we are more motivated to push through difficulties and achieve our goals. In order to break out of our routine, we force ourselves to do new things.

Create routines and practices that will help you succeed.

Mental fortitude is merely a habit that can be cultivated through regular, purposeful effort. These practices help us form self-affirming convictions and attitudes that strengthen us to face and overcome life's most insurmountable challenges. Of course, it requires effort to form these routines. It requires persistent effort over protracted time frames. Furthermore, it calls for putting oneself in perilous situations and figuring out innovative solutions.

When we work out, our muscles grow stronger. Constant tension, soreness, and exertion lead to muscular enlargement. Your mental fortitude muscle is no different. Every opportunity to flex and exercise this muscle is a must. The mental exercise of "working out" this muscle is useful, but actual physical practice yields far superior results. Do something that pushes your comfort zone just a little and builds up to it gradually. With time and effort, you will grow wiser and more capable of handling life's challenges. This leaves us with the question of what kinds of thought processes will make us stronger in the face of adversity. All right, let's check that out.

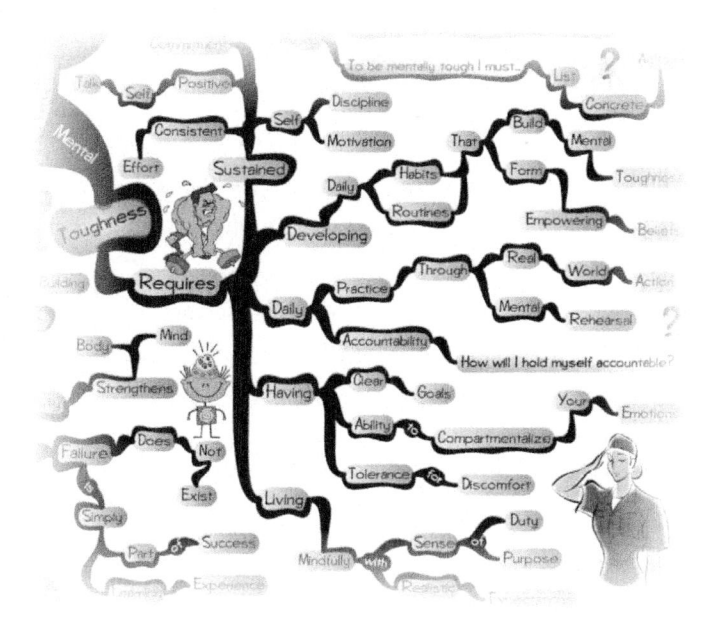

What makes some people more mentally resilient than others?

Let's look at the beliefs, habits, and ways of thinking that mentally strong people develop to get through life's hardest challenges.

What a Person with a Strong Mind Thinks

We act in accordance with the principles we have come to believe in over the course of our lives. These convictions can either propel us forward or hold us back. The truth is something that can only be known on an individual basis. This isn't the truth or the reality of the situation. In essence, this is why we put so much stock in our various systems of belief. If you put them to good use, they can get you through some of life's most difficult situations.

People with strong mental fortitude have a unique set of core beliefs that help them keep going when things get tough. The reason they're unusual is that few people choose to use them. That's why they can't handle life's challenges because they don't have the mental strength to do so. Using the first-person point of view, I hope to facilitate your internalization of these ideas. You'll need to read them regularly (multiple times a day) over the course of several months for the information to sink in. The next step is to put these convictions into practice, starting out slowly and working up to more ambitious goals. You must take ownership of them before you may use them. You can find a list of them below:

- I know that difficulties are fleeting and can be conquered.

- In my opinion, there is no such thing as failure. You can look at setbacks as nothing more than stepping stones to success. In other words, it tells me how I can improve my performance going forward, which makes me more efficient.

- I've learned that adversity makes me stronger in every way: physically, mentally, and emotionally.

- The more I take calculated steps toward my goals, the more assured I feel.

- Ultimately, I think there's a reason for everything. Everything that happens to me happens for a purpose that benefits me in the long run. Even though I have no idea where this road leads, I am confident that it will get me where I need to go.

- If I put in the time, energy, and effort, I think anything is possible. For this reason, I can never give up hope. It's possible that a major development is just around the corner.
- I think that good fortune follows those who are resilient in the face of adversity. When I apply myself diligently, show flexibility, and seize opportunities, the world rewards me. Success comes my way when I take charge and build a solid foundation of people to lean on for advice and assistance.

It should be obvious that there are other things to believe besides these notions. The list of tenets could be expanded upon indefinitely. Nonetheless, with just these convictions, you will have everything you need to muster the fortitude to face and conquer even the gravest of life's difficulties. Those traits alone will give you the courage and strength to take on any obstacle in your path.

Obviously, though, not everyone will agree with this. In reality, the majority of people do not hold these perspectives. Their unique set of convictions colors their perception of the world in a way that prevents them from progressing. Whether or not other people concur with these convictions is irrelevant. Whether or not they work for other people doesn't matter when you're facing the challenges that life always brings.

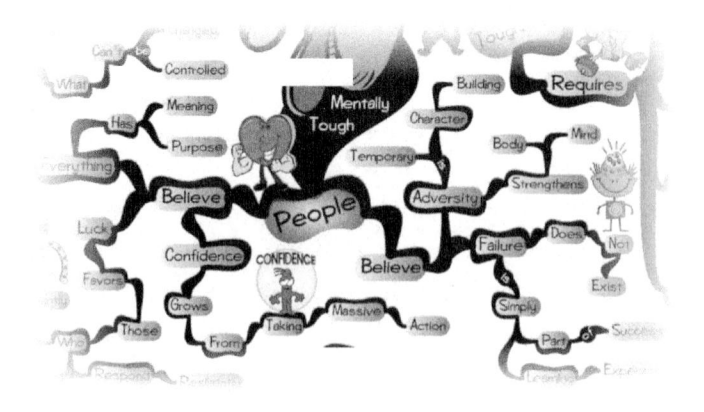

The Mentality of a Resilient Individual

Of course, a person's set of beliefs is only one part of their amazingly strong mind. Our ideas, beliefs, and linguistic habits, as well as the actions we take as a result, are the remaining pieces (habits). People with strong mental fortitude never blame others for their misfortunes. They don't point fingers, moan, or make excuses for themselves. They don't do the kind of catastrophic thinking that often ruins people's efforts.

Instead of complaining, they just deal with it and try to make the best of it. Making up excuses, blaming others, or complaining won't help you much. In the short term, it may improve our mood and our outlook on the situation. Long-term, however, it serves little purpose. People with strong minds are aware of this, and as a result, they are able to accept reality as it is. They let go of their attachment to outcomes they couldn't alter or improve upon and looked ahead optimistically. A sample question they could pose is:

- Why is this helpful, exactly?

- For what reason is this amusing?

- Exactly where could this lead?

- Where can I find a window of opportunity?

Tough-minded people believe that when one door closes, another one opens. They have faith that a chance will present itself to them at some point. Problems are unavoidable, so mentally strong people take a solution-focused approach. Because of this, they plan ahead to deal with challenges and difficulties. When trouble arises, they know that being ready will allow them to think more clearly and make better choices.

The difficulties we face in life are rarely simple. Not every contingency can be anticipated, no matter how well we plan. Mentally tough people are always eager to take in new information and use it to better themselves, no matter what challenges they face. They take on every obstacle with the enthusiasm of a newcomer and the determination of someone who believes they can never fail.

Naturally, blunders occur on occasion. Mistakes are inevitable, but mentally strong people don't let setbacks stop them. They change their strategy based on what they've learned from their past mistakes. They also gain knowledge from the mistakes of others, which aids them in preventing future, more expensive mistakes. It's a given that we can expect some degree of uncertainty in the future.

Mentally tough people embrace uncertainty and never take things personally, while less resilient people shrink from it and dwell on their bad luck, rejection, criticism, and mistakes. In fact, they use this fear to propel them forward in the pursuit of their objective. People with strong minds just get going when everyone else is worrying about doing things correctly. They rarely choose their timing carefully. Instead, they make the most of the present situation and accept whatever comes their way. Making the most of even minor successes is a driving force in their pursuit of greater ones.

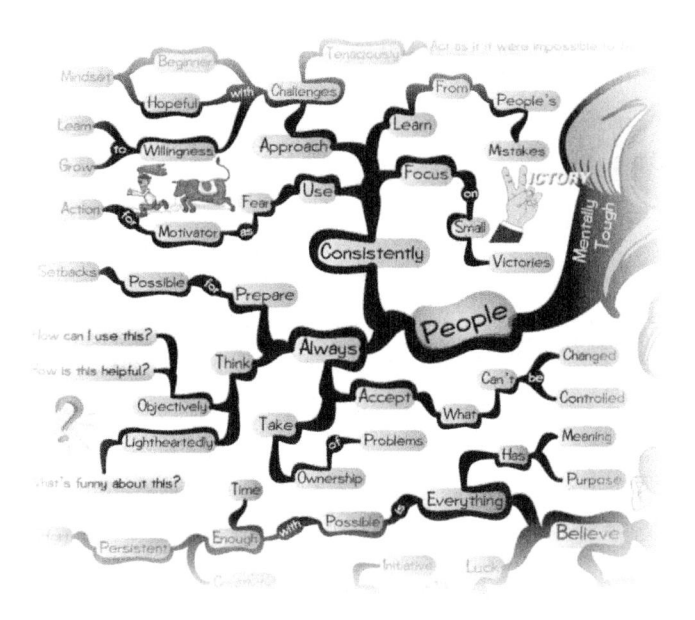

The Language of an Iron-Willed Individual

Individuals who are mentally strong use language as a motivator. They use the following methods to verbalize their optimistic thoughts and attitudes:

- Believe in me; I can pull this off...

- As for me, I know in my heart that I can do it.

- Don't stop making progress...

- Don't give up, no matter what.

- The answer is yes...

- This is something I am capable of doing...

- Someday I'll figure out a way to make it work...

These words serve as a source of strength even in the most trying of circumstances. What's more, they propel them in the direction of their goals. In times when life feels out of control and overwhelming, they help them maintain focus and motivation. A mere assertion, however, is not enough. They need to be paired with questions that can generate new perspectives and prompt course adjustments. Because of this, people with strong minds are always asking themselves questions to figure out how to solve a problem or make a situation better.

- What can I do to improve?

- What do I take away from this?

- How can I make the best of this unfortunate situation?

- How can I benefit from this circumstance?

- Is there something I can do here that I hadn't thought of before?

These kinds of questions open up the possibilities and encourage smart people to think about different ways to reach their goals. All this information points to the fact that the main characteristics of a mentally strong person are the language they use, the beliefs they hold, and their level of determination.

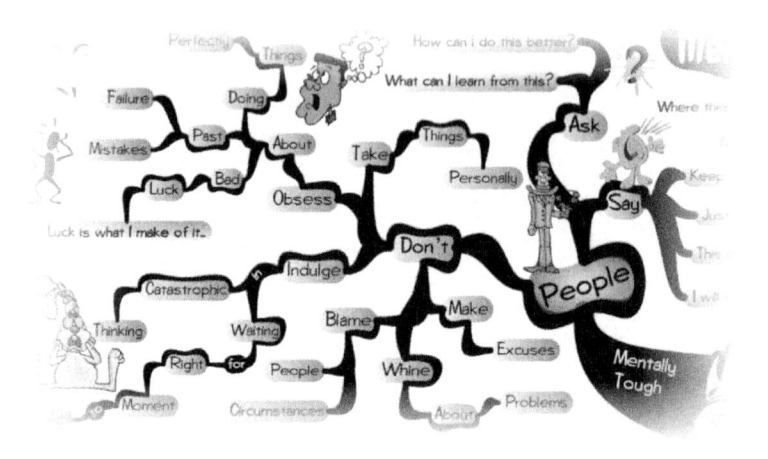

That's pretty much what it takes to build up the kind of mental fortitude that will serve you well when facing the inevitable difficulties of life. Developing one's mental toughness is a process that will take time and effort. It's remarkably similar to a muscle, which, like any other muscle, needs to be worked out and strengthened over time through consistent use. In spite of this, with time and effort, it can develop into a hidden superpower that will serve you well in the face of adversity.

Chapter 7

Tracking your Gains

Why it's a Good Idea to Keep a Fitness Journal

If you keep tabs on your body, health, and fitness, you can use the data to make informed decisions about your diet and exercise routine that will get you closer to your goals, whatever they may be. This information could help you or your doctor figure out if you are at risk for diseases like obesity, high blood pressure, or diabetes based on your body composition. These are a few general benefits of this kind of monitoring:

- Check your progress regularly.

- Evaluate the results of your workouts and diet.

- Motivate yourself to keep going.

- Develop wholesome routines.

- Evaluate the outcomes of your choices.

- Choose your next course of action with confidence.

- Get to know your physical self and zero in on what works for you.

It's difficult, if not impossible, to tell how much improvement you've made in your health and fitness without keeping track of the numbers.

- When you think back a year, how much heavier were you?
- Six months ago, at what depth could you squat?
- When you add a new exercise or alter your routine, do you see an increase in your strength?

The only way to find the answers to such inquiries is to keep track of your nutrition, exercise, and other bodily parameters.

If you use a tracking tool or even just a simple journal, you won't have to guess, and you won't be able to deceive yourself. It's hard to tell if you're making progress toward your goals if you don't keep track of changes. Physical growth is slow and subtle, making it difficult to notice on a day-to-day basis. Keeping a fitness record makes it simple to look back at past progress and evaluate it against current levels of fitness. Reading through your records will boost your motivation since you will be able to see the results of your efforts and appreciate how far you've come.

If you want to lose 50 pounds of fat or gain 15 pounds of muscle, you won't do it overnight, but with a realistic schedule and the right diet, you can achieve your objective. Habit formation is the process of doing the same thing over and over again until it becomes so strong that you don't even have to think about it. Keep in mind that the Eternal City wasn't constructed in a day, so if you run into difficulties along the way, don't give up and focus on your WHY instead. There are countless variables, from the most fundamental ones such as:

- Your caloric intake
- How often do you workout
- Your activity levels
- Desired goal

The following factors, albeit to a lesser extent, also contribute to this:

- Intensity of training
- Exercises you choose
- Rest between sets

If you keep meticulous records, you'll be able to spot patterns, pinpoint places for growth, and determine whether or not your initial strategy was too risky, not risky enough, or just right. The right plan is the one you can stick to; if you can't do it as written, don't do it at all and make adjustments as you go. You'll be able to take charge of your health and fitness in a long-term, sustainable way, thanks to the knowledge you gain from this information.

Methods for Monitoring Strength Training Results

Congratulations if strength training is already a regular component of your fitness routine. It's an essential part of every training program. In large part, this is due to the fact that using only your own body weight as resistance enhances muscular strength and force output. Strength training has numerous positive effects, but it's necessary to monitor your development. It's not like running or yoga, where you just end up more flexible and with more stamina.

Muscle mass goes down as you get older, so strength training is important because it fights this trend while also speeding up your metabolism. People can lose weight because they expend more calories. This is because the body responds to the strain by laying down new bones, particularly in the long bones of the spine and the extremities. This helps build up bone mass and either stops the effects of osteoporosis or even reverses them. The primary objective of strength training is to increase muscular strength.

To get the most out of your gains in strength and muscle size, you need to know when to lift heavier weights or do more reps. To accomplish this, just keep tabs on your development. Fitness professionals provide detailed instructions on the best ways to monitor your strength training sessions in order to aid you in achieving your muscle-building objectives.

Keep a workout journal.

Keeping a workout log is a simple and effective technique to keep tabs on the total amount of weight you've lifted over the course of your training career. In this manner, you can gauge your level of physical improvement. As we constantly put in an effort to improve our fitness, our bodies quickly adjust to the new demands. Thus, the body will stop responding to new challenges if we always use the same weights and training routines. The most common mistake I see individuals make at the gym is to repeat the same routine every week using the same amount of weight. Keeping a workout log, on the other hand, can encourage you to try new approaches to strength training. You'll be able to keep your muscles constantly challenged in this way.

Record the weight lifted and the number of repetitions performed.

Your exercise log is the perfect place for this. A second option is to keep track of your progress in your smartphone's notes area and update it after every workout. One objective method of tracking strength training development is to keep a journal of your lifting and aim to increase your weight or number of repetitions each workout for a period of six to eight weeks. If your gains have slowed or stopped, try increasing the weight by five pounds or the number of repetitions by one.

Check your body composition.

Checking the ratio of muscle to fat on your body is another good way to see how fit you are getting. Strength training allows you to simultaneously gain muscle and lose fat. The amount of fat in your body will decrease. Skinfold calipers and electric conductivity testers are common tools used in health clubs to estimate body fat. The direction of the trend can indicate whether or not you are making positive strides. Expecting to gain muscle mass means that your current weight may not be an accurate reflection of your progress. If you lose a pound of fat and gain a pound of muscle, your overall weight stays the same, but your fitness level increases. Stay cautious about putting too much stock in your body mass index.

Test yourself once a month.

Strength tests should be done regularly (every four to six weeks). Do fewer repetitions of an activity and keep track of your progress. Do reps with as much weight as you can while maintaining proper form. If you decide to repeat the process, be sure to evaluate your progress in relation to the first attempt. This way, you'll have hard data to back up your claim that your strength has risen.

Take a look in the mirror.

Focus on every arm, leg, and shoulder muscle as you take that selfie to record your overall fitness progress. When you first begin a strength training program, you may notice a more rapid reduction in fat around these areas. Because we always see the same familiar face, we don't always notice how much we've changed. The differences will be obvious in images taken four to six weeks apart.

Use a tape measure.

A tape measure is a simple, time-tested method that can be used to monitor your strength-training development. Take measurements of your shoulder, chest, waist, hips, legs, and arms using a fabric tape measure. You can track your progress and see any physical changes by taking new measures every four to six weeks.

Improving the Outcomes of Your Strength Training by Keeping Tabs on Your Development

Do you keep a log of your training sessions and check in on your development as you go? An important part of strength training is keeping a workout record, measuring progress, and keeping tabs on heart rate. Individuals can always know where they stand in their strength training program when they keep track of their progress. Having a fitness tracker allows individuals to monitor their development in a number of ways. That's true both in terms of appearance and supporting evidence, like a graph showing development. Next, we'll look at some of the best ways to track progress in strength training in more detail.

Fitness Journaling

Make an exercise schedule or fitness notebook and record your progress. A fitness notebook could contain a synopsis of each and every workout. This can be as extensive or brief as you desire for each exercise. The fitness plan could feature additional information not seen in a typical workout diary. There could be a bar chart showing your progress, a calorie counter, and heart rate information in this section. The greater the depth of the data, the more sophisticated the technology required to analyze it must be. This is where some people could find a fitness app to be helpful. Bodybuilders who are just starting out will see significant improvements in their strength in a short period of time. Your fitness and health can only improve if you keep a fitness notebook and use it to track your progress. Learn from past successes and failures. With this method, you may track the development of each section individually. Total volume and intensity, as well as sets, reps, and rest intervals, all boil down to numbers. A few examples of journal sections are:

- Exercises completed
- Workout duration
- Energy levels
- Stress levels
- Training volume
- Training intensity
- Number of sets
- Rest intervals
- Reps completed
- Time of day

Logging your workouts helps you determine the optimal workout frequency and duration. It also reveals your pre- and post-workout emotions and feelings on different days. Because of this, modifications are made to the approach to make it more viable going forward. The information you get now can help you improve your training sessions in the future.

Body Measurements

Taking regular measurements of your body is just as important as keeping a notebook when it comes to monitoring your strength development. The weight on the scale isn't the only indicator of success in the gym. While total weight is useful, the percentage of body fat provides more information. Aiming for a reduced body fat percentage is a common desire for the majority of people. There are a variety of methods for gauging fat reduction and overall body composition, some of which are more accurate than others. When it comes to determining one's body composition, a <u>Dexa</u> scan is among the most reliable methods. Although it's not the simplest or cheapest method, measuring fat loss is important. In addition to measuring fat, muscle, and bone density, the Dual X-ray

Absorptiometry may also assess a person's overall lean body mass. Using this method, you can see the changes in your body composition and muscle mass as you progress through your strength training program. Quicker methods exist for monitoring strength training development and body composition. As an illustration, consider the <u>InBody device</u>. Measuring progress toward goals on a monthly basis is an effective way to keep motivated.

Strength Testing

Building muscle requires a systematic approach, such as periodization. Instead of merely thinking about your workouts, it's crucial to take a step back and examine your overall fitness plan. Long-term preparation yields favorable outcomes. The major achievements are the cumulative results of months and years of training. One of the most important aspects of strength training is dividing the program into phases in which the gains made in the previous phase serve as a foundation for the next. Keeping a journal might help you keep tabs on the adjustments you need to make going forward.

By testing every eight weeks, you can monitor and assess your progress. You can easily determine what you need to do to improve. Your next round of training will be much more targeted once you have this information. Setting achievable, challenging objectives is much easier when you can see how you are doing. In the long run, success is more likely if you regularly assess your present level of strength.

Connecting the Dots: Monitoring Strength Development

Strength training would go nowhere without numbers to track improvement. Keeping a record of your progress can be useful in ensuring your own consistency. The benefits of these metrics extend beyond only strength gains to improved fitness as a whole.

You get information on

- Cardio and physical activity

- Your goals

- Exercises completed

- Sets, reps, and weight

- Energy and mood

- Mobility and stretching routine

- And more

Your confidence can be increased by keeping track of your training progress. You will develop better mental and emotional health in addition to physical health. It makes you more aware of the importance of maintaining a healthy lifestyle outside of the gym as well. This leads to decisions about how you spend your time and what you eat, both of which affect your health and happiness. Positive reinforcement is achieved through the examination of your exercise journal.

Conclusion

There are numerous advantages to keeping or gaining muscle mass. The health of your muscles, tendons, and joints affects your metabolism, hormones, and even mental acuity. Keeping your mobility as you get older is crucial to your health and happiness. Building muscle allows you to keep your independence in your movement well into old age. You have found a comprehensive, doable exercise plan in this manual. Muscle gain is possible with or without a gym if you concentrate on performing full-body workouts. This all-inclusive strength training guide places an emphasis on safety, and it does so by providing useful, accessible tutorials and illustrations that will lead you to a stronger, better you.

This easy-to-follow guide not only gives you useful information about how diet and exercise can improve your health, but it is also full of research that backs up the idea that strength training exercises can help you reach your fitness and weight goals. Many people agree that strength training is the most beneficial and effective exercise program out there. Though this book is primarily for gym goers, athletes, and seniors, people of all ages, sexes, fitness levels, body types, illnesses, and those just starting strength training will find it useful.

To live a fuller and longer life, you need to take care of your body and keep it in good shape. Regular strength training can help relieve pain from conditions as different as osteoarthritis, back problems, diabetes, and depression. Anyone looking to get stronger and leaner without shelling out cash for a gym membership will find this guide helpful. You can learn the proper and safe way to lift weights without the help of a personal trainer. This guide is a great resource for both sexes who are just getting into the habit of working out and want to know where to start. Learn how to get the most out of your workouts with the advice in the Beginner's Guide to Strength Training, which covers topics like safety, nutrition, and more.

Get into the best shape of your life at any age with the help of this book. If you're just getting started, don't worry; I've got you covered. I will help you get back in shape if you used to exercise regularly but haven't done so in years. After all, physical fitness is a key factor in continuing to take part in your favorite pastimes as you get older.

All the information in this book has been written with your age and safety in mind, and it's all presented in a clear and straightforward format. Follow this encouraging and informative manual on the path to a robust, well-rounded life. This book will help you get into the best shape possible, even if it has been years since you last worked out, by providing you with simple, step-by-step exercises that will help you reconnect with your body while minimizing the likelihood of injury. You need only participate; I'll handle everything else!

Printed in Dunstable, United Kingdom